# Battles of T

MW00454487

## By Linda McClure

ISBN 978-1-7388198-1-2 **(Paperback edition)**

ISBN 978-1-7388198-0-5 **(Kindle edition)**

# Dedication

Mom/Nana—1933-2020, love you, miss you, rest in peace.

To my son, my child grown into a man. My caregiver. My roommate. My friend.

Devon, I have no words to say how much I love you. There are no words big enough to say thank you. There are just not enough letters in the alphabet to say how proud I am, how impressed I am at all that you do and have done for me. With much love, Parental Unit, your mother.

To my family, those attached by blood and adopted.

# Contents

## PART ONE

## PART TWO

# PART THREE

## *2017—2018—Commuting to Alberta*

# PART FOUR

# PART FIVE

# Introduction

My story is complex and does not sit within the stereotypical 'box'. It is so far removed it's on another dimension. They diagnosed my epilepsy in 2015 at 49, followed by a secondary diagnosis of Psychogenic Non-epileptic Seizures in 2019. I'm one of the 30% who are drug resistant, anti seizure medications do not control my seizures. And I'm one of the 10-25% that live with both epileptic and non-epileptic seizures.

To be told you have seizures caused by your thoughts—hidden emotions trapped within screaming to get out—is unsettling. To have two types of seizures identical yet with different triggers adds another layer of anxiety—increasing the intensity of the vicious cycle you live in. You should be relieved. Thankful that therapy is the form of treatment, not drugs, and the only damage to your brain are emotional scars. But you're not. Thoughts of you're going crazy and it's my fault. I'm causing the seizures and thoughts of "suicide." It isn't a life. It's hell. An ongoing nightmare stuck in a war that will never end.

My doctors called me a mystery ... an enigma. I've had all the tests and procedures available. I've written this book to shine a light on the complexities of my chronic illnesses, the search for understanding, the whys and how comes. This book is for my fellow sufferers, the medical professionals and researchers, the curious, and family and friends.

I own the words written. The opinions expressed here are my interpretation of what I remember, experienced and journaled about. The facts of my journey are based on actual events as they happened, are not recommendations, medical advice, or 'how to' guide.

*Some names have changed, and others omitted to protect their privacy.*

# PART ONE

# Chapter One

## **The Beginning**

December 23, 2011: The office closed early to prepare for the Christmas holidays. After a round of hugs and well wishes and a quick change into yoga pants and a top, I grabbed my bag and headed out. The day was cloudy with a light mist, the type that showers the windshield like a light coating of Vaseline, smearing, and distorting your vision with each swipe of the wipers. It was still daylight, making the half-hour drive to the Bikram's hot yoga studio far more pleasant than most days.

Holiday shoppers were out in hoards, which reduced the number of students laying their mats down. My boyfriend Daniel had given me back my Zen zone with his gift of a Bikram's membership. I missed those days of sweating in a 40-degree room, the salty droplets running down my body. Hot yoga wasn't cheap. I hadn't been in years. A one-year membership cost $1,000, which we didn't really have, but Daniel felt I needed it and he made it work.

It was my third class back in my little *haven*, and all the old poses were coming back to me with ease—proud of myself and of my practice that day. The number of breaks when I laid down with my cold-water bottle on my forehead to cool me down were less than the previous two sessions. But towards the end of the class, I became nauseous and couldn't complete the final pose. Something wasn't right.

I came to in a waiting area surrounded by crying babies. Bored teenagers slouched in worn padded chairs, sporting cuts and bruises, looking bored and angry. A police officer stood nearby monitoring a group of three boys, one sitting with cuffs—glaring at the man responsible for his presence. My head was heavy, almost too much for my neck to bear. It bobbed up and down and side to side, unable to keep steady. My pupils dilated; vision distorted as I half sat in a wheelchair, a blanket tossed over me. Daniel sat next to me; his arm stretched across the arms of my chair to keep me from sliding to the floor. I wasn't sure where I was or why. How did I come to be in this room? I had been at yoga. Hadn't I? I had no recollection of getting home to bed, waking up the next morning feeling trampled, woozy, and confused. Daniel filled in some missing pieces from my mind.

"You had a seizure in the yoga studio. They called an ambulance and took you to the hospital."

I stared at him. My body felt the icy grip of fear and I froze. The memories of those moments escaped me. My mind was a blank. Empty.

## **Journal entry**

*Arnold from the yoga studio called. He was the one instructing when I passed out and had my seizure. Apparently, when I thought we were going into the final breathing exercise, I was about five minutes too early, which is what tipped him that something was wrong. He came over to me and tried to get me to stand up and leave the studio while still instructing the class, but I was totally out of it. My eyes were open. I was doing the breathing, but not responding to him. There was a nurse and a police officer in the class. I believe they tried to assist him in getting me out of the studio, but I was just like dead weight and they couldn't move me. As soon as he could, he ended the class and had everyone leave. The ambulance was called at some point as well. He mentioned I bit my tongue. Boy, did I ever! I have never had this happen before. Did the hot yoga for one-and-a-half years previously and I've never passed out or seized. The blood work, CT scan and ECG didn't show anything. It's possible it was a case of not enough food and water prior to class or my electrolytes were out of whack. I felt dizzy and nauseous during the last part of the class and I'd lain down for a while beforehand. I do not recall Arnold coming over to me, trying to lead me from the room.*

Christmas and Boxing day didn't exist. I don't recall who came for dinner or what gifts we received. I spent the days in my bed only rising to eat or use the bathroom. My leg muscles were like limp celery and my arms sore from the shaking. It took days for the drugs they used to pass through my system. My tongue, swelled to twice its size, was bruised, a black stripe running along one side. The chewing Arnold mentioned had been my teeth gnawing on my tongue.

Simple activities like eating, drinking, and brushing my teeth were painful. I was embarrassed, numb, and scared. The fear of what had happened, the thought of it happening again plagued my thoughts, being present one moment and then not filled me with dread. Not knowing what occurred, what I looked like, had unsettled me. The shift into a dreamless, vacant state, awakening confused and sore, was not an experience I'd like to repeat. Daniel said the doctor placed a referral to a neurologist to review my incident and determine the next steps. I returned to work after boxing day to cover the office until New Year's. The traffic was sparse, with the schools shut down for the winter break and offices closed. If it weren't for the stock markets being open, we'd be closed too, but someone had to be there to answer the phones and process stock trades. But that was rare and dragged out the days. At least the commute from Delta to Surrey, normally a half-an-hour drive, had taken only twenty minutes.

With the holidays after my seizure, I knew it would take a bit before I'd hear about the referral, but ten days into January, I hadn't heard a word. Another week and it'd be a month since they sent in the request. I needed answers but didn't know who to contact, so I booked time with my General Practitioner to find out what had been going on.

"Hello, sir. How are you? Did you have a delightful break over the holidays?" I slid past him into the exam room and perched myself on the table. Dr. Patrick looked younger than he was, still sporting the fresh look of a university student. The

Irish lilt in his voice was soothing, a pleasant melody that calmed my nerves. His clinic was more laid back than most. Located just across the train tracks and nestled amid older cottages and "monster homes" popular since the 90s, it had a relaxed, almost hippie-like vibe. They wore no suits or traditional white coats—street clothes with comfortable shoes lent a casual atmosphere, friendly and warm.

"Happy New Year, Linda. I'd ask how your Christmas was, but it's clear what you'd been up to." He settled himself on his stool, brought up my chart on his computer screen, and asked what he could do for me. I fiddled with the straps of my purse as I described what had happened, or what I could piece together. He made notes, scrolled down the screen for a page or two, took a deep breath, which he released as he swivelled on the stool to face me. I remember his soft brown eyes looking straight into mine, shifting to the door and back to me.

"How did you get here? I didn't see anyone with you in the waiting room. Did you come in a cab or by bus?" He frowned as he relaxed his back against the edge of the counter, his legs stretched out and crossed at the ankles to keep the stool from rolling. My hands stopped twisting and rubbing the straps.

I looked down at my feet, at my shoes, shifted my butt on the table, and waited. His question wasn't what I expected. It puzzled me why it mattered how I arrived at the clinic. I bit the inside of my lip and pursed my lips. Uncomfortable with the silence, I crossed and uncrossed my ankles. It was such an odd question and yet I felt guilty, like I made a major faux pas. Moments passed before I lifted my head and looked at him, brows up, the right raised higher than the other, and asked, "Why? I drove here, of course. Is that a problem? I don't understand the question."

"Yes, it is. You're not *allowed* to drive for *six months* after a seizure, and not until cleared by a neurologist. Were you not told this? Did no one at the hospital inform you of this?" His voice raised slightly, and his accent intensified, highlighting the concern reflected in his eyes. He pushed away from the counter and turned to the computer, tapping keys, and switching screens, reading through notes, scanning reports.

"Nooo. No one mentioned anything about driving. All they said was they'd refer me to a neurologist. I have heard nothing, which is why I came to see you. To find out what's going on." The breath I'd been holding burst through my tips, releasing some tension. He informed me that should I've had an accident and the insurance company reviewed my medical records; they could hold me responsible. He cautioned me to take it slow going home. Once there, I was to park the van and leave it. I waited while he checked on the status of the request with a neurologist. My gut told me there wasn't one. I was right, Dr. Patrick couldn't find one. He placed one himself.

I left his office in a daze. Not only was I not told about the driving thing, the hospital screwed up and didn't send a referral. I knew from past conversations with my Mom who had worked in a doctor's office that requests such as these from outside of the hospital weren't urgent and would go to the bottom of the list.

My fingers clenched around the steering wheel when I drove home, keeping the needle on the speedometer below the speed limit and staying to the right, letting traffic whiz by me, their horns blaring, annoyed at my slow procession during rush hour. My heart pounded and my arms and legs were tensed, frightened I might hit something or someone. If I had another seizure, the possibility that I might injure myself or others resulting in tragedy was sobering. The turn onto our street, passing the sloping lawn, fir tree, and pulling into the concrete stencilled driveway, had felt spectacular. My limbs took a few moments before turning rubber, my hands to uncurl and arms to drop to my leg. I was like melted wax that dripped and slid down a stick of tension—turning into a softened lump, unmoving as it cooled.

Unable to drive, I relied on the public transit. It was winter then, and the days were short. Commuting from Delta to work, a thirty-minute drive, took two buses and forty-five minutes. Walking along snow covered sidewalks and icy roads and parking lots was a challenge. I fell twice on black ice, tearing a hole in the pants of my suit. Not all the stops had covered shelters, and most were exposed to the elements. Sleet, hail, and rain drenched me as strong winds pelted my face and froze me from the inside out despite the mild temperatures.

While I'd waited for an appointment, I turned to Google. I called medical imaging clinics and labs to speed up the process. I'd thought if I got the examinations done while I'd waited for my name to move up the list—if I had all the work done ahead of time,—I could get in sooner. But one call from the doctor's office at the Outpatient Clinic deflated my bubble. It hadn't made a difference. The problem was only one neurologist read the reports, and because of the volume, it had overwhelmed him. The lady at the clinic had said it would've been a month before Dr. Edwards could've reviewed and provided a diagnosis, and another month to see him. By that time, I'd had the initial EEG (electroencephalogram) to detect any electrical activity in the brain that could've caused my seizures plus an MRI. (magnetic resonance imaging). The MRI was to determine if I had any physical abnormalities. I completed both at private clinics. Dr. Patrick had requested the EEG, but I was on my own to arrange for an MRI. Between my Mom and I, we found a private clinic in Vancouver and had paid to have it done. Within a month, I'd had the prep work completed—all I needed now was a neurologist to uncover the mystery of what had happened. I'd circled back to my original issue of seeing a neurologist. All that time and money had gotten me nowhere, but lucky for me, the private clinic had a neurologist, Dr. Dunne, who agreed to review my case. It was April, four months since my trip to the emergency room.


The resentment I felt towards others, especially Daniel, had festered. I felt trapped while those around me came and went. Relying on others hadn't sat well, and I became frustrated. The construction company Daniel worked for was busy. Overtime was expected, and he worked late and on weekends. That left me stuck at home doing housework and dealing with teenaged drama. Juggling the demands of a stressful job, handling the cooking and cleaning, and supervising unruly teens, only enhanced the negative emotions that swirled inside. I was tied to bus schedules and the generosity of friends, and I hated it and everyone around me.

To rule out the possibility of a heart condition, Dr. Dunne ordered a Holter monitor test. The lab technologist placed stickers on and around my chest and attached them to a recording device similar in size to a tape recorder. She'd given me a booklet with instructions on what types and how to log activities, times, and duration. I had to wear it for twenty-four hours.

I lay in bed that night with this box on my chest, the booklet and a pen, and a flashlight next to me on the nightstand.

It was 12:20am the first time I woke. I had to pee. I hadn't wanted to disturb Daniel, so I used a flashlight to enter the time and what I'd been doing in the boxes. The first time I got up, I'd almost dropped the pen as I sat on the toilet, juggling the flashlight in my left hand, while balancing the booklet on my knee. After each visit, it took a while to fall back to sleep, only to awaken from the discomfort of the monitor as it shifted. When I rolled to either side, the box had slipped along my chest onto my arm. If I tried to sleep on my stomach, it was like lying on a brick or flat rock. Despite my tiredness, I returned the monitor and my entries at the appointed time of 8am and then returned home for a much-needed nap. It would take another six weeks before I'd get an answer.

Daniel took the day off to come with me to hear the results. After three-and-a-half years together, supporting him through layoffs and job searches, coming with me was the least he could've done. I can still picture myself sitting in Dr. Dunne's office with Daniel on my right. A stack of papers rested in the middle of a cheap desk with a fake wooden top. There was very little in the way of decoration in the small room. The desk, three chairs, a waste bin, and a small table off in a corner with a small printer sitting atop. A framed certificate hung on the wall across from me, stating Dr. Dunne's credentials and where he'd trained. The remaining walls were bare, which amplified the dingy, windowless room.

"Hello, Ms. McClure. Thank you for coming in." Dr. Dunne edged behind me around the desk and took his seat. He placed a thin file folder on the desk, nodded a greeting at Daniel, and settled himself in the creaky chair. He shuffled through the pages he'd pulled from the file folder, his glasses resting on the tip of his nose. His mouth moved as his eyes scanned the words and his head nodded from time to time as he shifted from one report to the next. Daniel seemed unperturbed while I twitched and squirmed in my chair, craning my neck as I tried to read the words reflected in his glasses. His sudden movement had startled me when he'd looked up. Well. It couldn't be that bad if he was smiling, right?

"Really? Are you sure? Oh, wow." I grabbed Daniel's arm and squeezed. I hadn't any cancer, or an aneurysm, and I wasn't going to die.

"Yes. As far as your test results have shown, this has been a one-off occurrence. One of life's mysteries. A once in a million occurrence that most likely won't happen again." Satisfied, we left.

*I look back on that day and smile. It's a sad smile reflecting on the irony of the words he'd spoken and how much my life had altered since then. It's almost laughable.*

The days of getting up early. Travelling on the bus in the wind, rain, and snow and begging rides from friends - feeling stranded and alone. All of that would stop and life would resume as it had before.

On May 28, 2012, I received word. It was official. I could drive again.

# Chapter Two

## **Moving On**

Unbeknownst to me, that episode altered me. It wasn't just the struggles with a dysfunctional medical system and how hard it was to get answers. Nor losing control, the helplessness and sense of isolation. It was the state of my mind—how those sparking neurons had messed with my head. I wasn't the same person—I had transformed, and my relationships deteriorated.

An organized multi-tasker at work, I'd been geared for optimal efficiency. File drawers arranged and labelled allowed for the immediate retrieval of forms and notes. The desk was clutter-free–only the necessities required for that day's tasks covered the mahogany top. I liked order and cleanliness. My obsession with cleaning extended to all that encompassed me. From the car to home. My biggest hurdle was those who lived with me.

Daniel, his two kids, Mark and Jessica, and even my son, Devon, were the Oscars to my Felix. To arrive home to a kitchen littered with plates, cups and pots filled with remnants of meals, set my teeth on edge. Often it expanded elsewhere—

the living room, the basement and under their beds. It drove me insane. After the seizure, my compulsion intensified, and I'd convinced myself they'd done it to taunt me. It was a game to force me beyond my limit. Our house became a battlefield–it was me and Devon versus them, and it was my fault.

Daniel and I argued about the kids. Their laziness, how he thought I'd given Devon preferential treatment. And I'd respond with my resentment over the disrespect exhibited towards me by his kids, and so on. I did not know raising three teenagers would be so hard and how immature they could be. They weren't babies anymore, both Jessica and Devon seventeen and Mark fourteen. Almost adults in my mind.

"You treat my kids differently than Devon. You never rag on him as you do, Mark and Jessica. You overlook his digressions and won't offer my kids the benefit of the doubt," Daniel said.

My jaw clenched and a fiery heat rose from my belly, enveloping me, distorting my vision, and made it hard to breathe.

"If your kids worked with me and quit being such drama queens and if you didn't undermine me, stating you're on my side and then instructing them to ignore me, it wouldn't be as big a problem, would it?" I answered.

Daniel rolled his eyes, turned away and played angry birds on his phone. The conversation was an old one, and he didn't wish to examine it. I was dismissed. He would close himself off behind his invisible barrier and stuck his head in the sand, ignoring the issues, hoping it would disappear. The flaming discontent inside me spewed forth two weeks before the Christmas of 2013.

Daniel and I had been out and arrived home to a kitchen scattered with debris. A frying pan left on the stove a scorched sausage sunk into the congealed grease. Crumbs around the toaster spread across the granite to the floor. Half glasses of juice and milk stood in the sink. Plates and bowls rested on the counter above the dishwasher. The door open, and the racks empty. They left behind a slice of toast on the floor in front of the garbage can—peanut butter smeared down the front.

"Oh, for fuck's sakes!" Feet planted apart, my arms reached out, I motioned to the clutter. "Seriously? Come on, Daniel, that is ridiculous." Daniel stepped to the sink and started emptying the glasses, tossing the liquid down the drain, spraying the wall, counter, and faucet.

"Don't get bent outta shape. I'll tidy up your precious kitchen." Daniel retorted. His tone was demeaning and harsh. His movements abrupt and determined as he threw cutlery into the basket and jammed plates into the bottom rack.

"What're you doing? Don't clean this up! Get Mark to do it. We both know he created the mess. I can hear him downstairs. Get his ass up here." I stopped at the doorway, jabbed my thumb down the stairs to the basement. He was playing Call of Duty on the Xbox; I could make out the machine guns and soldiers. Both Devon and Jessica were working, so we knew the culprit was hiding downstairs. Daniel stopped, spun and glared at me, arms crossed, his eyes mere slits below his bushy brows.

"You just can't handle it, can you?" Daniel said. "This mess bothers you to no end, doesn't it? Everything must be done your way. And done on your time schedule. There's just no pleasing you. My kids can't do anything right."

I leaned against the counter and glared at the floor. He would not draw me into it. There was no point. He'd never listened. Couldn't perceive things from my point of view.

"Want ice cream?" I asked. I pulled out the Neapolitan ice cream pail from the freezer, propelled him out of the way, grabbed bowls, scoop and spoons and had waited. My reaction wasn't at all what he'd expected.

"Yeah, sure." Daniel responded. He shrugged and returned to cleaning. He loaded the dishwasher and tossed items into the sink filled with hot soapy water to soak. The clanging and banging he created as he'd gone around the kitchen had been deafening. I'd just remained there, silent, and scooped Neapolitan ice cream into dishes, careful not to send the chunks flying as I chipped away at the frozen dessert.

"Am I doing this right? Does this meet with your approval?" His breath oozed with sarcasm that filled my eardrum, causing me to stop. "What? Did I do it wrong? You going to wash up after me? Get it perfect?" Daniel bumped into me. The ice cream dropped to the counter, and I froze, holding my breath to keep from talking; annoyed and angered by his carelessness. With stiff, jerky motions, I wiped up the spill, and returned to dishing out the melting ice cream.

"Oh, no. What a mess. Oh my, you better clean it—*such a tragedy*." His hands waved around in alarm, covered his face as he danced on the spot, pretending it had outraged him.

"Oh, fuck off and cut it out, asshole!" I retorted. But he'd kept hopping on his toes, arms flailing, eyes wide, continuing on saying how terrible it was. Even today, I don't know how it happened. I elbowed him aside and resumed my task. When he hip-checked me, a mechanism clicked and my hand clutched a glob of ice cream from a bowl and fist raised, had thrust it into his face: smeared it all over, crammed it up his nose into his moustache and along his jaw.

"You bitch!"

His words snapped me out of whatever trance I'd been in and I hunkered in the corner by the back door, heart beating through my breast, eyes fixed on the melted puddle at his feet. I was physically sick. Stomach muscles cringing constricted the air flow. I was horrified. I could get furious, yes, but not to where I'd act out. As the shock wore off, I bolted along the hallway to our bedroom, ashamed of what I'd done. I slept in the spare room, curled up on the couch. The next day, I packed a bag and took off for my mother's. My actions had disturbed me. When I discovered Daniel had told Mark of our fight and the ice cream face wash, I seethed with rage. How dare he? Mark *had caused* the argument, and Daniel had no business discussing our disagreement with him. I was annoyed over my actions that I'd lost control. But with Mark knowing the details, how could I look him in the eye? I stayed ten days at my Mom's and refused to talk to Daniel. I needed time. If it hadn't been for leaving Devon behind, I'd have stayed away longer.

With the stress of my job and the chaotic turbulence at home, it was only a matter of time before I'd erupted. The atmosphere at home had worsened. The tension coiled up tighter and I couldn't handle it. I searched for excuses, avoiding home after work. I ran unnecessary errands, had drinks with colleagues, drove under the speed limit and chose the longest routes home just to delay the inevitable. It was then I'd started using the gym at work. It was a fully equipped gym accessible to those who worked there, and it was free. Twice a week, I went to release the stress and apprehension that coursed through my body. Most days I'd had it to myself. By 4 pm, shorts and a t-shirt donned, water bottle full, runners laced up, bag in hand, I buzzed myself in.

The months passed and our 'forever home' became a prison for me. It was not a refuge. Not a home and certainly not a place to relax after the pressures of a busy workday. The tension was heavy, thick, and strong. If Daniel's truck wasn't in the drive when I pulled up, I kept driving. It didn't matter where I went. All I knew was I hadn't the desire to walk through the front door. I never knew what I'd be faced with. A house full of teenagers, stoned, a kitchen counter littered with debris—music blaring. Devon spent more time away from the house, only coming home to sleep. He lived in his bedroom, only coming out to eat and use the bathroom. Daniel took on more and more shifts at work, stating we needed the money. When he was home, we avoided each other. Daniel spent more time with friends going out for drinks that extended into the dinner hour. Tired of holding down the fort and planning meals that no one showed up for, I hid at the pub. Listening to music on my iPod, I'd sit at the bar alone with my thoughts, sinking deeper into depression.

By then I realized my ties with Daniel had unravelled and the closeness we'd shared over the last six-and-a- half years had evaporated. The ongoing stress and theatrics weren't worth the effort. I wasn't happy and the only way to fix it was to sell the house and go. My decision increased the animosity and resentment that hung in the air. We were in a war zone and I was the enemy.

We'd listed in February 2014. When I told the gang at work, I'd whooped and danced around my office, laughing and crying. I stood up straighter, smiled more and the coiled snake in my stomach had unwound. The offer came in April and we removed the subjects in May. We had sold! It was such a relief—the freedom exhilarating. I could hear the birds, when before I only heard my painful cries. I saw rainbows where the storm clouds had been. My body floated through the days, feet barely touching the ground.

I located a two-bedroom, two-bathroom apartment near our family and friends. A newer four-storey condominium with shops below and condos above. An attractive design of rich coloured bricks and stonework, oversized balconies and patios. A rectangular pool of sparkling water that bubbled up in the centre and spraying over the edge of the fountain, showering the paving stones. Ideally situated, they constructed the condominium next to a mall. All the conveniences were just a few strides from our door.

On June 1, 2014, Devon and I moved into a top floor corner unit overlooking the entrance and fountain and a view of the mountains in the east. Sunshine filled the rooms through the floor to ceiling windows, blanketing the white shag carpeting, painted white walls and vaulted ceiling with sunlight. The kitchen opened into the living room, separated by a long island. A small dining nook was just large enough for a small dining table and four chairs. We loved our new home. The calm quietness provided that much-needed oasis after a hectic day we'd both been missing.

## **Journal Entry November 20, 2014**

*Another girl's weekend done. It amazed me how much food and alcohol we consumed, the late nights and dragging our asses out of bed the next morning with a skull three times the size it had been before you passed out. The day we headed home, my stomach had gurgled and swirled on the verge of erupting and my bowels were going to explode. The sensation enveloped my frame, created ripples from rear to front—part dread, part flu, but without the nausea or temperature. My vision distorted as though looking through binoculars backwards. Never had I experienced anything close to it before, and I blamed work stress and ignored them.*

It had been a rough nine years since I'd left Devon's dad. His death four months after we left, the strenuous relationship with Daniel and his kids, scarred both Devon and me to where our relationship deteriorated. With the stress we'd endured, I decided we required something to look forward to. We'd talked of a return trip to Disneyland for ages. It was a great time to do it. A few emails, a phone call or two, and we set off. March 2, 2015, we flew out. I booked a hotel closer to the park to see the fireworks better. We dumped our suitcases in our room, sorted out the sleeping arrangements, meaning who took the bed next to the air conditioner, then headed out into the warm spring breeze in search of food. It wasn't spring break in California–I had chosen a period where the place wasn't overrun with rug rats and baby strollers. We'd be in and out in a week. Our plan was to hit the rides and lands that we hadn't in our earlier two visits. And to end off our visit, we'd spend our last night at the Honda Center to see the Ducks play against the Penguins. We rode the California Screamin until we couldn't yell any longer. We toured the Lego store, sat in a bar, and gawked at a block of screens. Each one aired a different sport. We came home with suitcases crammed with hockey memorabilia, t-shirts and ball caps. The camera on my phone held photos of Disney characters and park attractions, videos of parades and fireworks. Refreshed and relaxed, we returned home to a fresh beginning–a restart or reboot to our lives.

Five days afterward, the warmth of the California sun was replaced by an icy fear of such size and far-reaching consequences that it had shifted the trajectory of my existence.

Daniel and I had met each other on weekends–on my terms. After six-and-a-half years, it'd been tough to let go. It turned out to have been an unwise and unhealthy choice on my part. We'd been to the pub for dinner and drinks. I recall little of that evening–teetering on our lofty perches amid pitchers of beer and dirty shot glasses. I know we made it home to my bed where I woke the next morning with a pain in my skull so powerful I thought it would shatter. A handful of Tylenol and a gallon of water had worked in the past, but this proved to be more of a challenge.

"You okay, Mom? Do you need anything?" Devon asked. He'd never seen me in such a state. Daniel had already taken off.

"Hand me those extra strength headache tablets and some water, please." I croaked from the couch. Buried in pillows and an ice pack balanced on my head. It hurt to talk, to move, to think.

"Here you go." He deposited the bottle and a glass of water on the coffee table, made sure they were within reach. A peck on the cheek and he headed for the door. "I'm heading out. See ya later."

"Thanks." I grabbed the pill bottle and glass as I battled to sit upright. "I'm going to lie on my bed and watch Netflix."

"Bye, love you," Devon called from the door.

"Love you too," I squeaked as the door closed and the lock clicked. I lay for a minute, my head pressed into my shoulders by the sheer pressure of misery. Extracted myself with care from my nest and shuffled over to the kitchen. I toiled to open the bottle at first, fumbling. I took two tablets out, popped them into my cheek, followed by a swig of water. Then refilled my glass and wandered into my bedroom, placed the glass on my nightstand and took up the Xbox controller and TV remote. I stopped in front of my dresser and peered at the Xbox. Never got the hang of it and Devon always had to set it up for me. I'd tried to envision the steps Devon showed me to access Netflix. The controller in my hand mocked me. Laughed at my ineptitude. After a few attempts, I had it up and working. When I look to recapture the events of that day, I'm standing in a fog–a real peasouper—the images from that moment are muddied. I assumed I headed to the toilet to pee before settling in to watch back-to-back episodes of The Good Wife.

# Chapter Three

## **Three Hours Later**

I could hear humming. Not sure what or where it was. My head hurt and felt fuzzy. My eyes fluttered open. Hesitant to look at the brightness. The movement was almost painful. I glanced around. White walls, a drape, or was it a door? Lifting my right arm, I felt a pinch. *Ouch.* Raising it to my face, I found dried blood and an IV protruding from my hand. *What the heck?* I went to touch it with my left hand, but it wasn't moving much. *What the fuck?*

My heart pounded in my chest as my eyes wandered about the room, trying to focus on every detail. The sterile white walls, ceiling and floor, the bed. An IV pole stationed beside the bed clicked every so often. To my left stood a machine, making sure I had a heartbeat. A clothespin type clamp closed around my index finger, confirmed I had a pulse, that I was alive, at least from a physical standpoint. I did not know what day it was—if it was morning or night. My body wracked with pain was too weak to move. My brain, dazed, confused and helpless.

"Good. You're awake." A woman stepped in, a clipboard under her arm, and came to my bedside. She wore pink scrubs with matching coloured shoes. A purple headband held back her long brown hair, letting it swing freely. She stared at the machinery flanking my bed, placed her glasses, which hung around her neck by a lacy cord of pink, purple, and white, on her nose and scribbled notes. I watched as her head bobbed up and down, transferring information from machine to paper, not saying a word. Finished with her task, she came to my bedside. "Hi, I'm your nurse, Karen." She smiled. Pulling out what resembled a fancy tire gauge, she leaned closer. "I need to take your temperature and listen to your heart. Is that ok?" I nodded and shrugged. What else could I do? They had me so tangled up in cables, tubes and wires, I couldn't stop her if I wanted to. Karen put her stethoscope away and turned to leave.

"Hey, can I have some water? Please?" My voice sounded small and weak even to my ears.

"Sure." With a smile and a nod, she slipped out the door.

The afternoon dragged on. Sleep was no longer possible. With no TV or phone, I resorted to watching the surrounding screens. When tired of that, I counted dents and scrapes on the walls and dots on the ceiling tiles. I was closing my eyes when the door opened, and a man strode in. Short and squat, balding and wearing spectacles too big for his face, making him appear bug-eyed. He stared at the monitors, walked to my bedside.

"So. Ms. McClure, is it?" he didn't wait for my response. "Good news. We're sending you home. We're confident that you're out of the woods, and we can release you." Consulting the clipboard he had tucked under his arm, he continued. "We will place a referral for you to see a neurologist. They'll be in touch when they've arranged an appointment. We called your son to come to pick you up." As he turned to go, I spoke. My voice was loud and more robust than it had been.

"No. I'm not leaving until an appointment is booked with the neurologist." He turned around. The determination in my voice shocked me. He stared at me, sitting straight up with my arms crossed. He saw the stubbornness mixed with desperation in the eyes that glared back.

"Yes. Well. Fine. Yes. I'll see what I can do." He backed away and slipped out the door. The shock of how I reacted replaced with a chuckle. Wow! This was the first time I had done something like this. I sat back, hugging my knees, nodding and grinning to an empty room—congratulating myself on sticking up for what I needed. I wasn't about to go through the hassle of tests and to see a neurologist like last time. It was this hospital that screwed everything up back then and damned if I'd let them do it again.

Taking a deep breath, I let it out long and slow, releasing the hot and heavy air that'd been weighing me down. *I guess I'm stuck here. Wonder how long it'll be for them to get me in to see someone.* The door opened again. This time, it was my nurse.

"Hello, Linda." She smiled, sympathy exuding from her pale grey eyes. "We've booked you to see Dr Terry next week. He's at the Outpatient clinic. Here are the details." She handed me a yellow piece of paper with an address, phone number, and a map. "Now. Let's take this IV out." She grabbed the gauze and surgical tape she'd deposited on my bed and shuffled over to my right arm. "Your son will be here soon. We instructed him to bring you some clothes. The paramedics ruined your shirt and bra when they were assessing you. I hope they weren't your favourites." She looked and sounded guilty. As if it were her fault. Such a sweetheart.

"That's ok. They're only clothes. Thank you." She moved fast, and before I knew it, she pulled the IV and affixed a bandage in its place.

"Take care of yourself, Linda."

The drive home, eating dinner, was a space of nothingness until I'd stepped into my room. No memories flooded back to me, only a paralysing sense of fear and anxiety. Dressed in my PJ's, I stood in the doorway of my ensuite. An invisible force held back my progress. I stared at the floor. *How did it happen?* My eyes shifted to the vanity. They wandered over to the doors and along the granite top. *Did I hit my head on the counter on my way to the floor?* My stare moved to the tile. Inspecting each grout line, I tried to summon a vision, a memory of something, of what had occurred. I think I recall going into the CT scanner, but not sure if it was an actual memory or if they'd told me about it. I was not aware of my surroundings until Monday morning—the seizure happened on Sunday and I wasn't released until Tuesday. There was no explanation to why it happened, only conjecture and assumptions. Whether traumatized by the event, Devon didn't want to talk about it. He went out—came home—found me, called 911, I went to the hospital, came home. End of story. The doctors figured I seized for a long time, and my symptoms would be like what one would experience from a severe concussion. My head felt wrapped in cotton batten, and I couldn't focus. To string words together and make a sentence was like a child whose vocabulary was growing.


I tried to piece together what had happened, but my mind was blank; nothing sprang forth. The events that took place sucked up into a black void. It ripped out a page of my life and tossed it away—gone forever. I lost a moment in time and left with a hollow space. Each time I entered the bathroom, I stood in the doorway, taking long, deep breaths before stepping into the room. Fear and anxiety were swelling up from my belly—a billowing flood filling every crevice, pushing to the surface. Taking it slow, I would stand at the sink, wash my face and brush my teeth—hands and legs shaking. Afterwards, I would collapse onto the bed, exhausted. The trauma of that day stuck with me for weeks. I couldn't be alone. Dev drove me to and from work, or I took a cab. The odd time a co-worker picked me up or dropped me off. On the weekends, I spent the day at my mother's while Dev was at work.

As I got further away from that day, my sense of humour resurfaced. I joked I was a 50-year-old babysat by an 82-year-old mother and a 21-year-old son. No one seemed to understand the impact it had made. I got the sense that since I survived with no long-lasting physical effects, moving on from it should be easy. I didn't have broken bones; I wasn't lame, nor were my movements hampered. It was inside that broke. My sense of wellbeing scarred beyond recognition.

## **The Teddy Bear**

March 26th, 2015, it felt surreal sitting in the waiting area. I was the youngest one there. Mom came with me for moral support. We sat amongst a crowd of wrinkleys, as my English cousin would say. Some more pruned up than others. I flipped through a magazine, glancing at the ads, not bothering to read the words. Mom had brought her Kobo and sat beside me. Her hand had caressed and patted my leg periodically. The door opened. An older gentleman, sporting the usual white coat, and with a scowl, bellowed,

"Linda McClure?" My mouth had gone dry, palms became sweaty and as I'd walked past him into the office, my legs had almost given out. I stole a quick glance as I passed him and took my seat. His voice was soft, and he spoke in a soothing and gentle tone. "I'm Dr Terry. How are you doing, Ms. McClure? You had quite a scare, I imagine." His look was soft and full of empathy. "Looking at the consult notes from the emergency room, it appears you had quite the seizure, young lady. Not to scare you, but seizing that long starves the brain of oxygen and can cause severe brain damage. You were lucky to come away unscathed. You're lucky to be alive."

I'm sure my mouth was a gaping hole as I stared at him, unable to move. Speechless.

"I want to point out that your bloodwork showed a high alcohol level. Are you a heavy drinker? Do you have a problem with alcohol?" His eyes bored into mine, probing my mind to extract the truth.

"Was her birth a difficult one? Were forceps used? Did you carry her to term, or was she premature?"

"No, my pregnancy was normal. No complications, and she was a few days early. Why?"

I sat there, my eyes moving from him to the window, to the floor and back again. My hands clasped to keep them still. He turned to me and continued.

"Have you suffered any head trauma? Or been in any car accidents? Any other seizures in the past?"

"No-" Mom began.

"Yes," I interrupted. "Well, no accidents, but I had a seizure three-and-a-half years ago. Back in December 2011." He consulted the papers in front of him, added some scribbles, and placed the clipboard on his desk. Scooting his chair closer, he continued.

"We'll do a series of tests to see what's going on. I'll order an MRI and an EEG. Once I've received the results, we'll have a sit-down and determine the next steps."

"How long do you think it will take to get these done? The last time we had to go to private clinics and had trouble getting into a neurologist. Lucky for me, Dr. Dunne, who reviewed my MRI, took me on as a patient. It was a nightmare and took months to get it all sorted out." My chest constricted at the thought of going through it all again—the frustration, the anger, while scared senseless.

"It shouldn't take too long to get in. I suspect you'll be back here in a month or two for the results." Thinking that was it, I gathered up my purse and coat and was putting my notepad away when his hand touched my arm. "I can't stress how important it is that you stop drinking. I mean it. No more alcohol. Ever. And no driving for at least six months." He squeezed my arm, then let go. "Can you promise me that?" A lump grew in my throat and tears pooled in the corner of my eyes. I took a small breath, savoured the fresh oxygen for a moment, raised my head and expelled the tense air from my lungs.

"Yes. I promise." He smiled, nodding his head. The seriousness of what he told me registered. I could have died. *Wow! Fuck me. Shit.* He said I could've had severe brain damage. I could be a vegetable lying in some hospital bed or institution.

"Ms. McClure? Linda?" Coming out of my inner self, I stood, turned to the doctor, who turned out to be human, shook his hand and turned to leave. "Don't worry; we'll figure it out.

See you soon." I nodded and smiled as I thanked him and left the room.

All I wanted was to get home. I needed to process things and allow it to seep into my disturbed brain. Knowing l couldn't jump into the van and drive off again gave rise to the same emotions as before. The sense of loss, a grieving for what I couldn't have, no matter how much I wished it. The weeks moved by as I ran through the same tests I had three years before. This time, I knew what to expect. The fear of the unknown held no power over me. This time I had the system working with me—not against or ignoring me entirely. The big difference was l could not get past how close I had come to death.

*How could this have happened again? Had there been signs I missed? Could I have avoided this?* The being inside me had changed. I wasn't the woman I had been. My essence had dried up and blown away as if a dandelion had gone to seed. I'd had more support from friends and family that held me up. It made testing, wait for another test, and more waiting, bearable. I adjusted as best as I could. Waking each morning to the brightness of another day. Going through the motions.

Showering, applying just enough makeup to smooth out the blotches and scars left from the chickenpox contracted in my thirties. Dressing in business suits, grabbing the purple quilted lunch bag, purse, keys and water bottle, careful not to wake Dev.

## **The Diagnosis **

Work was the only thing that helped shut out the voice in my head. Seizure—three hours—stroke–; brain damage; death bathroom floor. All these thoughts kept racing through my mind. Like an Indy car speeding around the oval, jockeying for position, trying not to crash and burn. I was now taking the bus to and from work. It was a short walk in plain view of others, should anything happen. My early morning trek took me past dark storefronts and the morning shift, loading orders into the delivery trucks at Save-On, and across a busy street to the stop. As I passed the vans, one fellow always had a kind word, his smile genuine, his laughter full of life, not forced.

"Well, don't you look nice," he said the first day I wore a dress to work. Each day, with a cheery voice and a smile on his face, he was there. Don was his name, but I called him my morning Save-On man. He boosted my ego with his compliments and was a great way to start my day.

As the weeks passed, I'd break down at my desk. Slumped in my chair engulfed in wrenching sobs, unable to focus. The sympathy of my coworkers faded, not used to seeing me beaten up. In the past, I would laugh and joke, always finding the silver lining to any storm that brewed overhead. I was a stranger to them now, someone they didn't know. I was in the middle of an episode when one of them popped in to ask a question.

"What's wrong? Hey, what's the matter? Come on. Get yourself together. You're stronger than this."

"I can't stop." I looked straight past her; my eyes blurred with a waterfall of emotion. Shaking her head, she threw up her arms and walked away. Exhausted, emotions raw, I turned back to my computer screen. It, too, was blank—black with swirling colours of ribbon dancing across the screen, mocking me.

Taking a deep breath and wiping my eyes, removing the makeup, I talked myself down off the cliff.

Dr. Terry ordered a sleep deprived EEG. It meant I had to stay awake throughout the night and *without* the aid of any caffeine. I arrived early at the outpatient clinic. I needed to keep moving around so as not to nod off.

"Hello, I'm Debra, and I'll be performing your test today." She was blonde with kind eyes and delicate hands. She showed me into a small room set up with monitors, a reclining chair and a set of cables resting on a metal table. Pulling a stool from the corner, she grabbed the electrodes and a bottle. She uncoiled the tangled mess. Grabbing what looked like a pencil crayon, she began drawing on my scalp. "This is so I can connect the cables to the right places." In no time at all, she had my head covered in 20 electrodes. A fluorescent tube placed above my head. A round light, off to the side.

"Ok. Ready?" Subjected to flashing lights and strobes, over and over. For half an hour, it went on, and nothing happened. No twitching, no shaking, my conscious state not interrupted. As far as I could tell, the test was a waste of time. "Alright, we're all done. Dr Terry will get the results in a few days. We'll be in touch. I've wiped off about as much of the goo as I can. Wash your hair when you get home. Take care." I opened the door, smiled and mumbled my thanks as I made my escape. Hair sticking out everywhere, looking like a porcupine.

I washed my hair in the kitchen sink, being careful not to splash watery goo everywhere. I wouldn't step into my shower without Devon at home. The trauma from that day hadn't left me, and it took all the courage I could muster to enter the bathroom. Giving up the struggle of brushing out the bits of remaining glue, I stretched out on my bed to catch up on those hours of blissful sleep I lost. When Daniel and I had bought the house together, I'd kept my townhouse and had rented it out. When I left Daniel, I hadn't known what I wanted or where I wanted to be, so I took out a two-year lease on a condo to allow time to think.

That May, I'd sent the lease renewal to my tenant. I hadn't expected the response I'd received. Her mother was ill and required help, and she'd given notice to vacate. My stomach dropped ten feet when I had read it. It was the last thing I'd needed. The lease I'd signed didn't end until June 2016. I couldn't afford to pay both mortgage and rent. Now what? Would they allow me to break the lease? Oh, man. Do we need to move again? My insides collapsed on itself—a pricked balloon losing air and crumpled. Do I sell my townhouse?

My seizure—work—being on my own. And now this added to the pile. I was like a stake pounded into the ground. With each fresh crisis, the sledgehammer sent me down. My body and mind were sinking further with each strike. Every blow crushed my spirit, splintered it into pieces. But I was fortunate. My landlord agreed to my request, and we moved mid-September.

## **The Results Are In**

All the tests completed; it was time to hear the bad news. Am I dying? Dr Terry's greeting was anything but gruff as he waved us in. Mom and I took our seats after we exchanged the usual pleasantries. He turned to his computer.

"We've got all the results and based on what we can see; it looks like Mesial Temporal Sclerosis." The screen blinked and produced what looked like an x-ray. Leaning forward, I peered at an overexposed black and white blob. He pointed at the image, moving his finger as he spoke. "This is the MRI image of your brain. This area here is a scar on the right side temporal lobe." Letting that sink in, he turned in his chair to face me, leaving his finger on the screen. "That scar, we believe you were born with it." Eyebrows raised, my look shifted from the blob to him and back again.

"But they did an MRI in 2012, and nothing showed up. The doctor had said it was normal." My eyes darted back and forth, but couldn't focus on anything. I'd just sat there. My chest and shoulders had collapsed. Breathing was difficult. I'd not known what to think or say. He thought a moment, fingers steepled, tapping his lips.

"It was possible that the scan wasn't at the right angle. Or cover enough of the brain to capture it."

"So, what does it mean?" Mom asked, while scribbling notes.

"It means you have Temporal Lobe Epilepsy and need medication to control your seizures. I'm going to place you on Dilantin and Keppra to start. We'll try these out and see how you manage. There are a lot of side effects you may experience. If you can't tolerate them, there are other newer epileptic drugs that we can try." He ripped off two pages from his pad and handed over the prescriptions. "You can fill this downstairs if you like." His smile was genuine, his look kind, full of empathy. Standing, he took my hand, helped me up and said, "One more thing, no more alcohol. I mean it. No more." I'd nodded, mumbling my promise to obey. "I'll see you in about a month." We shuffled out the door like a pair of zombies.

I jumped when his voice boomed out, calling for his next victim. But he wasn't the gruff old bear he portrayed. He was a big marshmallow inside. I didn't understand the situation or grasped the reality I now faced. Arriving home, I flung off my coat and shoes and grabbed my laptop, fell onto the couch. I talked to Google about Mesial Temporal, what's it and epilepsy,

Dilantin and Keppra. With my feet up and a cup of tea to keep me company, I scoured the internet.

I'd kept my pills on the bedside table so as not to forget taking them. My morning routine now composed of getting up, taking my pills, washing and dressing, packing up my breakfast and lunch, then off to work. The process repeated at night. In amongst our purging and packing, I'd paid another visit to Dr Terry. Since the discussion was about changing my meds, I'd brought my sister Margaret with me. She was a Nurse Practitioner, been a medical professional for over thirty years. It'd made sense to have her there.

The discussion had been short and sweet. Dr Terry reviewed the merits of the two different drugs with Margaret as I sat and listened. Margaret had done her research and peppered him with questions. She knew her stuff and had done what I'd hoped she would; remove the decision-making.

"Ok, Linda, we're switching your Keppra to a newer drug called Lamotrigine." He handed me a prescription. I glanced at the words, couldn't understand BID and the other Latin terms used. "We'll see you back here in two months to see how you're managing."

"Thank you, Dr Terry," and turned to go.

"Remember, no alcohol."

"Yes, sir." I gave him a big smile as I headed out the door. On my next visit, I was in a wheelchair.

## **Journal Entry May 2015**

*I'm now on anti-seizure meds and must live with the uncertainty that 'it' may happen again. If it does, will it be worse? My heart raced when thoughts of the next one being even more severe washed over me. I'd sit with eyes squeezed tight, gulping for air, hugging myself tight, frightened I'd become a vegetable and not know who Devon is, or end up in a coma or die. Thank God for my family. I have an outstanding group of friends. They've all been checking in on me. The daily phone calls, coffee and lunch dates, helping me with errands, reduced my feelings of isolation and loneliness. I am blessed to have so many people who care about me. Dr. Terry said they'd found a scar on my brain. I now have a seizure disorder (epilepsy). I'd just been fortunate not to have had it earlier in life. Need to reduce stress, get plenty of rest, eat, and no alcohol (ever)—life-changing shit.*

I kept to myself, hung out at home and watched Netflix or sports. I stopped using the gym at work, opting for the one in our apartment building. All I wanted was to plug in my iPod and escape. I didn't want to socialize or talk about work. The minute I arrived home, I would change into my workout gear: shirt, shorts, socks and runners, and headphones. Grab a towel, water and my yoga ball, then head down to the gym in my building. Most times, I had the place to myself. No fights over the treadmill by the window, nor scrounging for weights or waiting for the bike or an elliptical. It wasn't a large room, tucked away in the back of the building. Bushes surrounded the pathway outside, leading to the windows and glass door had limited the amount of daylight. In July, I hired a personal trainer and between that and my morning Save-On man, I'd felt good about myself. Despite the interaction I had with coworkers, clients, friends, and family, I had been lonely. I'd been sleeping well but felt tired and listless, isolated and alone. Stuck at home, even though there were buses I could have taken to almost anywhere I'd wanted to go, but I couldn't bring myself to leave the five square miles of my hometown. My anxieties had trapped me within a cage of my own making.

## **Journal Entry June 5, 2015**

*One hundred and two days more, not quite halfway there—the entire summer to get through before I can drive again. I think weekends are the worst. No reason to get up to do anything; most of my friends are busy with their own thing. Hard for me to call up people and say, 'I'm bored, come out and play with me.' All I do is go to work—clean, a few workouts, watch Netflix or play on the computer. I'm bored.*

As the weeks went by, I experienced those milder flu-like symptoms like I'd had back in November 2014. They'd had persisted through December and into January, and February right until my seizure in March. It wasn't long before I discovered that those turbulent sensations were actually seizures. Experiencing a repugnant smell, déjà vu, (feeling you've been somewhere or done something before) or jamais vu (the sense of unfamiliarity–surrealness), flickering lights, hearing things, numbness and nausea were types of seizures called auras. Not everyone experienced them, but I had.

*[Dictionary.com definition of 'A Wave' - disturbance on the surface of a liquid body, a sea or a lake, in the form of a moving ridge or swell. - any surging or progressing movement or part resembling a wave of the sea.]*

The physical sensations that washed over me I'd described as 'Waves.' A rushing feeling that overtook my body, making me reel in the strength of its uprising. A heaviness in the pit of my stomach that churned around and around–heating as if rubbing two sticks together. Every nerve in my body tingled-jumped inside my skin. The churning tightened in the depths of my belly and rose into the chest. Then, like a huge

Wave, it would crash over my head and overloaded my senses to where I'd almost

passed out and then recede, leaving a burning lump.

# Chapter Four

## **Plunged Into the Depths**

### *August 2015 BC long weekend. Sailing Trip to Sucia Island with Margaret and my brother-in-law, Barry.*

Four months had passed with no significant events. Margaret felt I needed a break and planned a sailing trip for the August long weekend. She and her husband, Barry, took me out on their sailboat to Sucia Island just off the coast of Washington State. It had been a sunny day with a wonderful breeze. We backed out of the slip and motored past the other vessels. The only sounds were the rigging clanging against the mast, the seagulls calling out to one another, and the chug-chug-chug of the engine as it moved the 36-foot floating home across the rippling water. It had been a wonderful, relaxed weekend filled with fresh air, hikes, and card games. Margaret and Barry had treated me like a queen. I was served coffee and breakfast in bed and wasn't allowed to prepare meals or wash dishes.

Wind blew my ponytail hair about my head; deflecting off my shoulders into my ears and whipping my cheeks. I looked out across the whitecaps. Point Roberts was a bump on the horizon, a molehill of land among green water and blue skies. Then it hit. A queasy sea sickness in my gut followed by a smell so putrid its description had no words. Looking back now, I can only describe it as a mix of sewage, rotten meat and compost all mingled together, filling my senses, overpowering all else. My stomach overwhelmed me. I'd felt the heaviness and nausea rise and washed over me. It made me want to vomit. I'd thought I had eaten something that hadn't agreed with me, that the smell was rotten remains of a fish. I'd assumed a trip to the head below would've solved my problem. In reflection, it only complicated it.

I'd just finished when Margaret had called out to me. Orcas were breaching. To witness that would've made the trip perfect. I recall exiting the head and bumping into Margaret in the galley. She'd taken one look at my face and grabbed me.

"Linda, you're having a seizure," she stated and turned me towards the banquet seat, forcing me to sit.

"No, I'm not," I had argued that I'd felt fine, that she'd been wrong. I wasn't having a seizure.

"Lie down. Stay there," was the last thing I heard. Margaret and Barry told me afterwards they got approval to dock at the coastguard's station. How the paramedics guided me from below deck up and over the side to Margaret's car. Although I was unaware of my surroundings, I still responded to simple commands.

Cleared across the U.S. border to Canada without having to stop, we sped to the waiting ambulance. Deposited inside, my unconscious body strapped to the gurney bounced along the highway.

I came to in a room on a bed that wasn't mine, housed in a place that wasn't my home. The weeks spent in the hospital blurred. Being awakened each morning and during the night didn't allow for a good long stretch of sleep. It didn't matter, as I spent many hours dozing during the day. The nurses' station was just outside my door. They had moved me down the corridor from the first room they'd placed me to one across from the nurses' station. Easier to monitor me. I was in one of the new towers of the upgraded neurological ward at Sullivan Memorial Hospital. The sterile white walls were scuff-free and the linoleum floors still had a glossy sheen. The heavy wooden doors and cabinets were of blonde maple with chrome handles that reflected the harsh fluorescent lighting. I believe I had my own bathroom equipped with a toilet and sink. My memory has faded, but there could have been a shower too. The small window facing north overlooking a busy highway, towers, apartments, and a bridge had not escaped the touch of vandals leaving their mark. Scratches etched deep into the glass distorted the view. Past patients so bored had made big swirls and circles in the glass. Deep grooves following the same path went around and around. If drawn on paper, the pen would have cut through, leaving a flapping hole weakened by the continual pressure.

As my strength grew, I shuffled to the ledge and peered out through the lines at life which carried on without me. My world was now limited to temperature and blood pressure checks twice a day. Nurses delivered pills before breakfast and dinner, the dosages and names altered almost daily. I filled the time with books, crossword puzzles, and music. I wasn't a stranger to hospital beds, to being confined within stark surroundings, visited by strangers whose job it was to keep me alive and well. But that time was different. I'd never spent over five or six days in hospital except for my appendectomy and the birth of my son. We planned those, and I knew what was going to happen and wasn't afraid. Now, I was in a room that wasn't mine, eating food prepared by some unknown cook, deposited on my table on a chipped plastic tray. The bed wasn't worthy of a one-star hotel, and the pillow and blanket may as well have come from a dumpster, discarded by its previous owner as they lost their usefulness years ago. The days passed and folded one into another. Friends and family supplied me with puzzle books, novels, treats, and the odd real coffee. I spent many hours in a semiprone position listening to music. It was my only escape, better than sleep. The melodic tunes kept the reality away. Sleep brought night terrors where my inner self forced me to face the situation and played it over and over, like a recording looping repeatedly with no off button. I felt helpless, like an injured animal caught in a trap, the jaws keeping me from escaping.

Although I saw nurses and doctors each day, sent for tests and a multitude of vials filled with my blood, it didn't seem they were doing anything to correct my situation. I was under observation; they held a magnifying glass over my bed. Peering into my head while scratching theirs. I was a prisoner to science. Those waves of sensation passing through my neural network continued despite the drugs. My mental state deteriorated, as did my body. My senses became distorted. I heard a song by The Who that no one else could. It came from the ceiling, not my iPod. It played on and on, without pause. My vision, already impaired on the left side from the seizure, produced ghostly images. It happened after an orderly delivered my lunch. He'd deposited my lunch on the table, grabbed the breakfast tray, turned, and headed towards the door. I'd turned to thank him, but froze. In the doorway was just the outline of his body. A glowing type aura like an overexposed negative filled the frame, but he was at the nurse's kitchen on the other side of the hallway. I'd thought I'd seen a ghost. An icy fear spread over me; goosebumps popped out like hives. I pressed the call button.

The next morning, I'd thought someone had hacked my phone. The icons doubled in size and then disappeared. In my mind, a virus had taken over and was eliminating my only connection to the outside. My heart pounded, increased by the force of blood that pumped through my veins. I didn't know what I could've done to stop it. My hands shook, and all I thought was I had to call Devon. I stumbled to the nurse's station and begged them to use the phone. When they placed the handset into my hands, I'd cried. I remember pushing the redial button over and over until he'd answered. I'd woken him up, but I'd been desperate to tell him of my predicament.

"Mom, slow down. What're you trying to tell me?" My panicked voice tried to tell him that someone had hijacked my phone, and was deleting my apps, taking over my phone. The words tripped over each other as I rushed to get them out.

"Mom! Stop! No one is taking over your phone. It's ok. Here's what I want you to do. Take the battery out and put it back in again. Keep your phone off till I get there, ok? Do you understand? Look, I gotta go. Love ya, see ya later." Before I could react, he'd hung up.

"Linda? Hello Linda. Hi dear. We need to get you back to your room. Come on, yes, that's right. This way, that's it." Nancy, my nurse, had stood with her hand out. She gently took hold of my arm and guided me across the corridor into my room.

Once she was sure I was safe in my room, Nancy headed back to the nurse's station. Drained, consumed by my emotions, I dozed off. The arrival of breakfast interrupted my rest, but not for long before my head slipped to one side. The lab techs took blood as I laid there, completely unaware that vampire Joe had crept in and out. A touch on my shoulder roused me. Gentle shaking opened my eyes. I stared at the figure lurking around my bed.

"Hello, Ms. McClure, I'm Dr. Dondel. I see we have you on several medications. Phenytoin, Lamictal, Keppra. Let's get another CT and MRI. I'll see about when we can get those done, oh, and some bloodwork."

I looked at him as if he were the village idiot. Even in my numbed state, I knew he was wrong. My meds had changed. I was on four, not three. I checked them regularly with the nurses—driving them nuts. I checked my notes. The CT was happening today and bloodwork? Could he not tell by the wad of gauze taped to me that Dracula had been? I said something, but he'd gone. Never asked how I was doing. I picked at the remains of my breakfast, glancing over at the window in between bites.

The White Coats, as I dubbed them, did not instil the belief I'd be okay. It'd been two weeks and my daily visits included a doctor who'd seemed disconnected and disorganized. With my meticulous note taking, I tracked what tests they performed and any adjustments made to my meds. Dr. Dondel would show up and spout off orders for tests I had already completed, would discuss medication changes that had been in effect since the day before. Obviously so busy, he hadn't reviewed my chart, and it showed. He became known to me as Dr. Dindledorf. It was a name I created to describe individuals that no other words could. Almost three weeks passed before help arrived as a White Knight.

*[Throughout my stay, a weekly rotation of doctors (hospitalists) was assigned to my care, Dr. Dondel, aka Dindledorf, being one of them.]*

They brought in an occupational therapist to determine if my seizures had any adverse effects on my brain functions. To test my cognitive ability, they asked me to complete a worksheet. Questions like; what animal is this? Which of these pictures are of fruits? Count from 100 backwards to 70. Draw a clock showing 11:15., and so on. All questions that any adult could answer with ease, but for me, it was a challenge. The concentration and focus needed to complete these had drained me. My head hurt. My eyes ached. I was exhausted. I'd just got comfortable with my flimsy sheet and thin blanket wrapped around me when Dindledorf appeared.

"Good afternoon. I see you've had your CT. We need to find out when the MRI will be. I don't see any reason to change your meds; we'll keep them the same for now." He stood at the end of my bed, glancing around without looking at me.

"I've had my MRI, and my meds were adjusted this morning."

"Oh, I see. Well, right then, we'll carry on and see how things go." Still not looking at me, he turned and left the room.

I sat and shook my head. Will he ever look at my chart before coming in? Settled back under the covers, I resume my attempts to escape for a few hours in deep slumber. But my eyes wouldn't close. Sounds from the corridor drifted into my room and I couldn't shut them out. Frustrated, I sat up and started scribbling in my notebook. Too many things raced around my head to let me doze off. What are they doing about me? Anything? I'm laying here attached to three different machines; fed drugs to keep me from seizing, taking my blood, sending me for tests, drawing clocks and pictures, all for what? I don't know. And then this dumbass doctor who doesn't seem to know what's going on. I knew what pills I was on, and what tests I've had better than he does. And I'm the one with mental issues!

I'd had a follow-up scheduled with Dr. Terry at the end of that week and assumed they would cancel it with me being in the hospital. Margaret said he saw see me when I first came in, but that was two weeks ago. I think. I'd finally drifted off when my phone rang. It was my sister.

"Hey."

"Hi. Quick call. You're all set to see Dr. Terry tomorrow. The time's been moved up. You're going in the hospital transfer van. Give me a shout if you have any questions. Sorry. Gotta run. Take care." Click.

With the arrangements in place and untangled from a myriad of cords, wires and needles, they wheeled me down to the ambulance bay. I hadn't bothered to dress. In my housecoat and slippers, my escort wheeled me straight into Dr. Terry's office.

"My dear, I'm sorry. I had no idea you were still in the hospital. How are you doing?" My mind, still foggy, was dormant, like a bear in hibernation. I managed a weak smile and shrugged as if to say, I'm alive, I guess. "It appears things have not improved; have escalated, in fact." I sat still. The fear from deep down had sent shivers throughout. His chair squeaked as he turned and placed his hand over mine. A soft sigh escaped as he looked into my eyes. "Your case is quite challenging, I'm afraid. I spoke with my colleague, Dr. Edwards, and he's agreed to take over." My heart sank to my toes, my chest tightened as I held my breath. I didn't want to lose Dr. Terry. He'd been like an uncle. Or an older brother to me–looking after his little sister. It took a moment or two before I could respond.

"Ok, if you think that's best. When do I see him? Now?" I straightened as if to get up.

"No, not now. He'll see you in the hospital later today or tomorrow. He'll take good care of you. I promise. You're strong. I'm confident that you'll get through this." Patting my hand, he rose and opened the door and motioned for my chaperone to fetch me. I'll never forget his parting words. "Goodbye and remember, no more alcohol." It still makes me smile. I would miss him. Grumpy, old man, my ass; he's a marshmallow inside — a teddy bear in a grizzly costume.

Because I'd lost muscle mass, they assigned a physical therapist to me. My stamina had to improve before they'd consider my discharge. That and I'd had to prove I could cook and feed myself and finish my cognitive therapy.

As promised, Maria came with a student in tow. She'd wanted to try something different. She placed the chairs next to my bed, the table between them. She'd gone to fetch some supplies when the nurse came to do the morning vitals. She'd barely stepped into the room and stared at the display.

"What's this?" she asked.

"I'm having a tea party."

She gaped at me, concern spreading across her features. Just then, Maria waltzed into the room, supplies in hand.

"Oh, sorry, is this in the way?" The nurse looked so relieved. I burst out laughing after she'd hurried out.

"What was that all about?" I told Maria what I'd done. She chuckled and began setting up the table. "Okay, let's get started. You sit here."

"Sure. No prob."

After lunch, I was introduced to Stephen, the physical therapist. He had me walk down the corridor and negotiate a short flight of stairs. After three weeks in the hospital, my only activity had been to and from the bathroom. I had to prove I could function at home. That I could prepare meals, use the stove, wash dishes, and feed myself. After a few days of stretching my legs without falling down, Maria escorted me down to a kitchen. It was a full set up with pots, pans, and food. I gathered the ingredients for a pasta, used what vegetables that hadn't turned to liquid, set the table for two and cleaned up. Maria was pleased with how I'd handled myself, but my legs were not. Once back in my room, the exertion and strength it'd taken to stand, move between the fridge, counter and sink hit me. I slept until dinner time, not stirring until shift change and my morning vitals.

I turned 50 during my vacation at the hospital — no surprise party, balloons or big dinner out. I'd received my regular fare served up on a plastic tray. Visitors were kept to a minimum, as I couldn't handle the stimulation. Devon showed up with a card and gift in hand.

"So, it takes me being in a hospital for you to get me a gift?"

My life had been a series of nurses and lab coats that wandered in and out, sprinkled with visits from family and a friend or two. And then *'he' walked in.*

## **The White Knight **

"Good morning Ms. McClure, I'm Dr. Edwards. Dr. Terry mentioned I would come to see you?" Standing next to my bed, he smiled down and held out his hand. He was much younger and taller than Dr. Terry. He had brown hair cropped short with a hint of grey showing at the temples. His smile was genuine, his eyes gentle and kind. He had a relaxed way about him—a calming effect. His voice was friendly and soothing, and professional at the same time.

"Hello. Can you tell me what's going on? I've been sitting here, and no one's doing anything, and I don't know what's happening. What's wrong with me?" Tears of frustration, fear, and anger threatened to overflow. I grabbed the Kleenex box, but it'd been empty. Instead, I used my blanket to sop them up before the dam broke. His look was sincere and filled with empathy.

"Here, can I have that?" He pointed to my notebook. I nodded and handed it over. He sat on the end of my bed and started scribbling and drawing pictures. "Sorry, you feel like we've done nothing, but a lot is going on behind the scenes." He turned the book around so I could see what was on the page, and with simple words, he explained what they knew so far. I didn't understand any of what he said, but felt better he was there and taken the time to talk with me. He stayed for over half an hour, going over his notes so I could comprehend the situation. As he spoke, he patted my leg. I felt reassured that everything would be ok, and he was there to look after me. My body relaxed and released the tension at my neck and shoulders. It'd been a comfort knowing *something* was going on, although I hadn't seen it. He'd arrived on my fiftieth birthday and it was the best birthday present I'd ever received.

An entire month gone—three weeks drugged up in and out of reality and released to my mother's care for 24-hour monitoring. My cage had only moved; the observers from lab coat to doting parent—hospital bed to a futon, mass-produced canteen slop to actual food. Among all of that, I had been moving back into my townhouse and I hadn't finished packing before the sailing trip—my intention was to complete it after the long weekend. As my Power of Attorney, my sister Margaret handled the paperwork for the Medical Employment Insurance and Long-term Disability applications. And she dealt with my tenant. Family and friends completed and arranged the packing, cleaning and painters.

I had arrived in the hospital on two anti-seizure meds and left on four.

I saw Dr. Edwards a week after discharge and Margaret came with me to help navigate the muddy waters of the medical system and the bureaucratic red tape—my second set of ears. My brain was still experiencing aftershocks. Waves of feelings rushing up from my gut and whooshing over my head occurred daily. These were Auras—a seizure—a warning signal.

*[Aura: An unusual sensation such as unprovoked fear or a sense of déjà vu, a strange taste or odour, or a rising in the abdomen similar to being on a roller coaster. An Aura may present itself prior to a temporal lobe seizure, but not everyone has auras, and some who do may not remember them. They are the first part of a focal seizure before consciousness becomes impaired.]*

My stamina was non-existent. I slept nine to ten hours a night and napped every day. Life had changed little from when I was in the hospital. The only difference was better food and no visits from Dracula seeking my veins.

Dr. Edwards's office was sparse. I sat on the edge of my seat, hands gripping the armrests, waiting for the bad news. Margaret rested comfortably on her chair, pad and pen ready.

"Ms. McClure, I want to send you for Video EEG monitoring at Victory Regional Health Centre. They'll trigger some seizures in a controlled setting and catch it all on video. You could be there for upwards of a week." He turned to the computer screen and began typing.

"That's a good idea. So, would surgery be an option?" Margaret asked. The two of them discussed the merits and pitfalls of temporal lobe surgery and what testing we'd require beforehand. I didn't comprehend what they said. I'd felt like an outsider watching and listening in on a private conversation held in another language. As we left, I forced a smile and thanked Dr. Edwards, my White Knight, for taking the time to see me. I wanted to ask more questions, but I hadn't known what to ask. So I said nothing, and we left—my head like a bubble wafting in the air with no destination and nothing to tie it down.

Those first few months after my seizure, Margaret had spent many hours completing forms. My disability insurance had a ninety-day waiting period and meant applying for medical EI to provide a small pittance of funds to help pay my bills. It had been nowhere close to enough, and I'd no choice but to accept help from Mom. I hated it. Unable to work and with no sign of if, when, or ever I could work, we applied for the Canada Pension Disability. They declined me. According to the Canada Pension, my condition was not disabling and would not affect me long-term. It became obvious they knew little about epilepsy and its effects. With Margaret's help, we drafted a rebuttal. To help my cause, she had me prepare an impact statement explaining how my life was affected.

## **Impact Statement to CPP**

*Since my seizures in March and August 2015, my life has changed drastically. I have always been a cheerful, active, positive person and coping with these obstacles has been difficult; both physically and mentally. These challenges, combined with the side effects of my many medications, have altered my outlook on life. I have always been an individual who was organized and in control. I made plans, had to-do lists and goals and objectives that I wanted to achieve. Because of my inability to work and to drive, I have had to make numerous adjustments to my life. I now have to rely upon others to accomplish normal activities that I was previously able to* *accomplish on my own. With so many unanswered questions, the ability to plan and set goals is not an option. Since I can no longer drive, I have sold my van. I have no extended medical benefits to help offset the costs of my medications (approx. $170-$175 every 2 weeks). I have a cleaner to help out and my groceries get delivered. I have to rely upon family members and friends to run errands and get to doctor appointments.*

*I now have cognitive/short-term memory issues and get confused easily. I have to limit exposure to stimulating situations as it causes seizures. I have to limit my outings and can't go to movie theatres, concerts, or amusements parks due to the bright, flashing lights, strobes, loud sounds and rapid movements. I can't have planned activities on consecutive days. I need down-time in between outings so as not to get overstimulated and require daily naps as I fatigue easily. I cannot go swimming or take a bath without supervision due to the chance of drowning should a seizure occur.*

*I am waiting for my admission date to the seizure investigation unit in Vancouver to undergo EEG/Video Telemetry and to determine if I'm a candidate for neurosurgery. I will be away from family and friends and the emotional support they can provide. All the tests, the waiting, the unknowns have had a huge impact on my emotional state of mind which, in itself, triggers seizures. There is no cure. There are no guarantees that neurosurgery will work or if I'm a candidate. If my seizures cannot be controlled, my quality of life will remain as it is. I thank you for considering my application.*

*Sincerely,*

*Linda McClure.*

Their decision was reversed. And they approved me.

Writing my thoughts and feelings was how I coped. Throughout those months, and even with my family's support, I felt alone. No one could understand what I was going through. No one could relate to the fear I had over another event happening. What if the next one succeeds in its quest and kills me? Or leaves me brain dead on life support? I had no control over them, and I couldn't stem the worries and fears of the unknown. The endless answers to the same questions I asked time and time again, my refusal to listen to the voice of reason and the help offered was wearing thin. The negativity exuding from me was overpowering—a stench so bad it drove those closest to me away. Those around me lost patience.

My memory hadn't improved. It was weird. Stuff from a long time ago came easier to me than recent events. Things had to be repeated before they sunk in. Poor Margaret. I couldn't remember everything she'd told me. Moving from Medical EI to disability, and the whole CPP thing, confused me. I was convinced I'd go back to work soon, and it was all so unnecessary.

"Linda. You're not going back to work anytime soon. You've got to face the facts ..."

"But I could. I need to. I can't afford not to... I—"

"Stop it! You're in no shape to return to work. The side effects of the medications alone wouldn't allow you to perform as you did. Face it. You've got to be patient. Let's get these tests done and see what happens. Okay?"

Margaret and I sat at the dining room table poring over forms, making lists of my bills. It was a conversation we'd had many times since I'd gotten home. She was tired of placating me, of constantly reassuring me it'll all work out. I'd get the surgery and be back to normal. To my 'old self.' I was told to trust her and not worry about everything. She had it covered.

And Mom. My refusal to take her money—to feel like a charity case—drove her around the bend. It was all she could do to look after her baby girl. She worried about me. But they couldn't understand. Here I was, a fifty-year-old woman, a single mother with a career in the investment industry who couldn't handle her own money! I was a failure.

## **Journal Entry September 29, 2015**

*So now I'm 50, alone again, back in my townhouse, and diagnosed with a seizure disorder. Now what? Since December 2011. I've now had 3 seizures. March 14, 2015, and August 3, 2015. I don't fit the "mould" or the "box," so I am a bit of a puzzle for Dr. Edwards. Too many unknowns, too many "rocks to turn over" (as Margaret would say.) Lots of great friends, an outstanding family, but I still feel alone.*

*I keep trying to find a reason, an explanation to why this is happening to me… There aren't any… it's just the way it is. I have no control over my brain and when it short-circuits. The meds help to control things—but in my case, not entirely.*

*Sometimes I look back and wonder, why did I bother trying so hard to do anything? Why bother trying to improve my overall health? I get the fact that my life could be way worse. I could be dead; I could be severely brain-damaged or have a physical, debilitating disease. I could have cancer, Parkinson's, Alzheimer's, etc. etc. But what is it I need to do to be happier? Healthier?*

*What if the pills don't work? What if surgery isn't an option, or it doesn't work? What kind of burden am I going to be to my family? Can Devon handle all this? I don't know… no one does.*

## *Journal Entry October 11, 2015*

*I am now off work for who knows how long and am struggling with not knowing what's in store for me. My seizures are not under control, even with four different drugs, and further investigation is ongoing. That I will end up going down the surgery route is scary as hell. On top of all this and the emotional roller coaster ride, I'm feeling so alone. I have support from my family. Margaret, and her medical knowledge, has explained all the medical jargon I don't understand, and Mom has helped me out financially while I wait for the Medical EI to start. I never did like asking for money and especially don't now. Any option to decline had been taken away. I've missed that special someone to hold me at night when the fears, the tears and the overwhelming emotions come forth.*

## **Journal Entry October 16, 2015**

I've continued to have waves. All depends on what I'm doing. Being around too many people and too much stimulation still triggers them. Even with the increased dosage of the Lamotrigine. As of today, it's up to 100 mg twice a day.

I took a cab down to White Rock beach. I needed to be down there to help clear my head. I did okay until I walked along the stores and waited at the bus stop to go home. The constant movement of cars, noise, and people was a bit too much. I started to feel sick; like a wave was coming on. It actually didn't hit until after I got home—after a nap.

Being down at the beach was good, though. I need to continue with that; I think. It may help.

I know I've made progress since being in the hospital, but am not back to normal. There's no timeline, no definitive 'end' or answers. I'm having a hard time dealing with this. I like to know what's going on. I like to plan. I'm not a go with the flow—go with the moment type of person. I make lists, I like to *organize, I like control—I don't have any of that & it scares me, frustrates me.*

## **Journal Entry October 28, 2015**

*That odour has reappeared—five times since the 16th. A very slight odour seemed to be starting earlier today—but not 100% sure.*

*I have not been booked for the EEG & Spinal Tap re-do. I've called twice—nothing yet.*

*And to add to everything, the seizure investigation unit had a neurologist leave and have placed a three-month hold on new patients. Even though they received my referral at the end of September, I'm on hold. More waiting.*

*Saw my occupational therapist yesterday. She's referred me to the social worker for Cognitive Behaviour Therapy.*

*My Lamotrigine is now up to 150 mg, but the waves and odours still increased. Not sure why? Will mention this when I see Dr. Edwards.*

*I've been more emotional the last week or two. Feel like nothing is being done—having that hamster on a wheel feeling—going nowhere.*

*I'm having a hard time trying to be motivated. I tire easily. Sitting around doesn't help. I'm having a hard time looking for the positive in all this. I don't want to come across as a 'victim' but come on, haven't I been through enough already? I don't know what the future holds for me. It's scary to think about. I'm hoping all that I'm going through will lead me to a happier life.*

## **Journal Entry November 6, 2015**

*I sat the other day & added up all the waves & odours I've had since discharged on August 25, 2015. About thirty waves and eleven odours. On a positive note, I now have an appt at the Seizure Investigation Unit but not until July 5, 2016 (eight months from now). I have placed myself on the cancellation list.*

*Still no re-scheduled Spinal Tap or EEG.*

*I hired someone to come clean every two weeks. This should help reduce some of my stress.*

*I met the social worker, Sara, who helps patients with Cognitive Behaviour Therapy. I got more out of my one session with her than I did with that shrink I saw earlier this year. And it's free!*

*She said to try applying my strengths and abilities I use in my job to manage the seizures and uncertainties. She felt that based on my organizational skills and ability to strategize—I could come up with ways to 'damage control.' I have a lot of determination once I have a goal in mind.*

*On a good note, I did manage to walk all the way down to the beach and a couple of blocks along Marine Drive. That took me about forty-five minutes.*

Two months went by, and no word from Victory Regional. Dr. Edwards advised Neurologists were leaving, and the one remaining wanted to retire. It would be years before I'd get in. They only had two beds to service the whole province. Margaret and I sat in Dr. Edwards's office listening, wondering what would happen to me. I stared at him, then over at my sister, shocked that such a prestigious institution was falling apart. I shook my head. So lost in my thoughts, I hadn't heard Dr. Edwards at first. Margaret gave me a nudge to bring my attention back to the room.

"I'm going to place a referral into the unit in Calgary for video telemetry."

"What's that?" I interrupted.

"Let me explain. Video telemetry is where they perform an EEG and record it on video. You've had EEGs, so that wouldn't be any different. They'd glue the electrodes on your head as before, but this time you'd be on video, twenty-four hours per day." He stopped and gave me time to digest what he'd said and then continued. "They have some of the best neurologists trained in epilepsy and seizure disorders. I did part of my residency there. They have four beds, so the wait shouldn't be long." In the car driving home, I tried to absorb everything. Calgary? I've never been there. Who will stay with me? How long would I have to wait? Brain surgery? *Holy shit. Wow!* I wanted to crawl into my shell and hide. Emotionally and physically drained, scared, and overwhelmed, I laid down on the couch and with the cat as my blanket, fell asleep.

While we waited to hear from the seizure unit in Calgary, Dr. Edwards had me back for the spinal tap. Epilepsy isn't the only cause of seizure disorders. Tumours, strokes, cancer, brain inflammation and autoimmune diseases, such as N-methyl D-aspartate receptor encephalitis [NMDA] a condition in which the immune system attacks the brain and could trigger seizures. To check for autoimmune diseases, we had to withdraw spinal fluid and send it off for testing. Since my seizures had started later in life than was usual and had escalated so fast, he wanted to rule out all other options. If there had been a simple treatment I could've undergone and made it go away, he was determined to find it.

I lay on the table in the fetal position with only a gown and my underwear. The room was chilly. The pressure of the needle piercing the skin wasn't any worse than having blood drawn at the lab. But as he poked about, trying to locate a gap in which to pierce the cord, a stabbing pain shot down my leg. He'd hit a nerve. Dr. Edwards had tried his best, but he failed. No matter how much I tried to open my spine, to coil myself like a snail's shell, he couldn't reach the spinal cord. We had to try again using the ultrasound. Weeks later, guided by the image of my spine on the screen, he'd extracted the fluid.

2015 was a horrible, stressful time. The previous ten years hadn't compared to the emotional turmoil I went through, adjusting to a life that'd spiralled out of control. I had always been that person to find a silver lining in the darkest of clouds. I laughed at life and the obstacles it placed in my way. I was strong and determined. If I didn't like something—I would change it. If I couldn't move it, I went around it. When challenged, I pushed back. I was the victor in my battles—won the wars 99% of the time. This time, I couldn't fight back. This disease, this demon, as I became to call it, had taken over my soul, rendering it into little pieces. 'Can you help me?' wasn't part of my language. Being in control and planning every move ingrained in me—part of my DNA. To have that taken away left me stumbling in the dark with nothing to hold on to—no glimmer of light to guide my way. It made me feel weak—a child who couldn't perform the basic needs of living. The pent-up anger unleashed itself on those around me. No matter what they did to help, I saw it as them pitying me, which only increased my rage against what I had lost. One minute I was clinging to anyone who could steady me; the next, I was shoving them away. Margaret, Mom, and Devon took the brunt of my split personality. The desperation and fear heightened my senses, sometimes clearing the mist, other times fogging up my vision, creating a distorted view. Combined with the myriad of mind-altering drugs, it was amazing I could see, or hear, anything at all. I lived on a seesaw—one minute carefree with the sun shining on my face; the breeze ruffling my hair. Then the next whack crash. I would land with a resounding thump, falling off the seat, sending me flying. Back and forth, my emotional state altered. Fear, anxiety, depression, anger, and resentment towards the changes forced upon me, and guilt. Guilt for what I was putting my son through. Guilty for having to ask my family for help. Guilty for ignoring and declining invitations from friends. I thought I was causing it all; that it was a lie, fake, and I was to blame.

# Chapter Five

## **Waiting**

The months spent waiting for my inaugural visit to Calgary were tough. I knew what I had, but still no clue where it would take me. My journal was the one thing that kept me on this side of sanity and a step or two away from utter despair. The new year started, and I'd received the first of many calls from Calgary.

"Hello Linda, I'm calling from the Epilepsy Clinic at Foothills Hospital in Calgary. I want to let you know we should be able to fit you in within the next three weeks. I'm sending some information in the mail for you to read and will be in touch once we have a date." She had to slow down a few times so I could write it all down.

"Is this for my consult?"

"No, we're bringing you straight in for monitoring. No consult. I'll be in touch in the next few weeks. Take care."

I stood in the kitchen, elbows planted on the counter, my breathing shallow, eyes wandering about the room, looking for something to focus on. I knew this day was coming, but I wasn't ready. I didn't move—my brain, at a standstill, as was my body. A *few weeks?? No consultation? What the heck? Can I do this*? A week later, a thick envelope from Alberta Health came through the mail slot and landed with a thud. It took a while to read through the pamphlets and enclosed letter—even longer to grasp what it all said and to understand what preparations were necessary. I needed clothes that buttoned or zipped up in front, nothing that went over my head. Slippers, housecoat, toothbrush, toothpaste, shampoo and conditioner. Medications for before and after my stay. Books and crosswords, laptop or tablet, a change of pyjamas and clothes. Not too much stuff, mind you, as the rooms are small. 'Prepare to be bored,' it said. 'Confined to your room except for trips to the bathroom. No showers allowed, only sponge baths. The average stay is 7-10 days but could be more.'

Rushing along the sidewalk after my cut and colour, I hustled to get over to the bus stop to head home. If I missed that one, I'd have to wait 30 minutes for the next. B-r-ring/buzz B-r-ring/buzz. Crap.

"Hello?" I stopped to focus on the call. I had to stand still and look at the ground so as not to get distracted.

"Hi, can I please speak to Linda?"

"That's me,"

"Hi, it's the Epilepsy Clinic at Foothills Hospital calling. We've got a bed available in the seizure unit on Monday or Tuesday. Are you able to make it then?" Ok, take a deep breath. Let it go.

"Uh, yeah, I think so. Um, can I call back? I'm out, and I need to check with my sister. Someone has to come with me to get there." My hand trembled. The lining of my stomach shook like a piece of paper caught in a breeze.

"Right, yes, you're from BC. Ok, I need to know by tomorrow morning at the latest. I left a message with the details for your sister. If I don't hear in time, you must wait for the next one. I hope to hear from you soon. Bye, Linda."

Oh shit. My fingers fumbled on the touchscreen, trying to locate Margaret's number.

"Hey, kiddo. We were talking about you. Did you get a call from Calgary?"

"Yeah, that's why I'm calling. The lady said Monday. I need to be there on Monday. But I have to let her know because I didn't know if that would work." My words jumbled out as if I had finished running a race. I felt panicky, overexcited.

"Where are you?"

"At the mall heading home. Why?"

"Stay where you are, and I'll fetch you. Bring you back here to talk."

Margaret, Barry, and I sat around their dining room table - strategizing. I had to be in Calgary before February 8th. We decided the best course of action was to go on the Sunday.

"Barry will take you, spend the night and come back Monday. We'll get the tickets. Mom is paying, so don't worry about it." I slipped down in my chair, crossed my arms, looking down at my feet. I wasn't about to argue, my brain too muddled up, tired and feeble to care.

Barry and I flew out of the smaller airport in Abbotsford. It wouldn't be as overwhelming for me with the hustle and bustle of the larger airport in Vancouver. I always enjoyed flying—soaring above the clouds, leaving the earth behind—amazed at the patchwork quilt the landscape created. We were waiting in Calgary for our luggage when the dam broke. The emotions took hold of me like a volcano spewing its innards. Tears spilled over as I sobbed deep down from the depth of my soul—my chest spasming. Barry let me unleash the pent-up feelings in silence. I don't think he knew what to do. I had the bottle cap screwed back on when the luggage arrived on the carousel. We'd booked a room in a hotel in downtown Calgary thirty minutes from the airport and just a twenty-minute drive to Foothills Medical Centre where the seizure unit is located. We'd sat in the lounge eating burgers and fries and watched the Super Bowl on the large screen TV. Barry and I, both football fans, hadn't let our trip stop us from watching the last game of the season. It'd been a long day for me and, emotionally exhausted, I'd fallen asleep early.

Barry had left on the Monday as planned. He'd headed out earlier than I'd expected - he was eager to get back home. He'd left the number of where I was to call and left the room. I stared around the place, feeling lost and alone. I didn't know what to do with myself, so I made the beds, tidied the bathroom, and gathered up my belongings as I went. I'd dumped out my suitcase, repacked and reorganized what was already organized. Eventually, there'd been nothing left to do. I was ready to go, but it was too early to call. *Oh, what the hell.* I grabbed the phone and dialled.

"Hello? Yes, could I speak to Mary? I don't know. I was to call this number. She's a nurse?"

"No, no one here by that name. I've been here 25 years and never heard of her." I dropped the receiver to the desk, moisture building around my closed lids. *Now what? I'm in a strange city by myself. No one I can call to help.* Taking deep, slow breaths, I scrolled through my phone, looking for the number Mary from the Epilepsy Clinic had called me from. It'd taken a bit of searching, but I'd eventually found it, jotted it down on the pad the hotel provided and dialled.

"Good morning, Foothills Medical Centre. How may I direct your call?"

"Um, yes, I'm looking for the Seizure Unit? I'm supposed to call to find out when I go in?"

"One moment, please." The voice was pleasant enough, more helpful.

"Good morning, Epilepsy Clinic."

"Hi. It's Linda. Am I to come into the seizure unit today?"

"I'm sorry? Linda? Linda, who?" Oh no. Not again.

"Um, Linda McClure. I've come from BC. I'm supposed to call to find out…"

"Yes, Linda, right? Glad you made it. Can you come at 2 pm? Check-in at the main desk and they'll tell you where to go. We'll see you later. Bye," Click. Silence. I was alone again and I couldn't just sit there twiddling my thumbs; so I grabbed my bag and headed down to the lobby. There was a Starbucks coffee bar tucked away down a long corridor off to the right of the reception desk. February wasn't a month for tourists, so the lineup hadn't been long, only one person ahead of me. He only ordered a regular coffee and was gone in minutes. I was next.

"Good morning. What can I get you?" The Barista asked.

"Hi. Um. Can I get a Venti Caramel Macchiato and a bacon breakfast sandwich?"

"For here or to go?" There'd been a table for one left off to the side and up against a wall. Exactly what I wanted.

"Oh, for here please." Two minutes later, I sat with my coffee and sandwich, feeling like an outsider. The only hustle and bustle were from those dressed in suits with briefcases. As the customers ebbed and flowed, no one gave much thought to a woman that huddled over her table, with tears streaming down her face and the odd whimper escaping her trembling mouth. *Screw it. I can't sit here.*

# PART TWO

# Chapter Six

## **February 8, 2016—Seizure Unit—Foothills Medical Centre, Calgary, Alberta**

I arrived too early and had over an hour to spare. I purchased a juice and a muffin from the coffee shop even though I wasn't hungry but needed to pass the time. People were milling about the open area. Some worked here, and others were visiting, or were patients like me, waiting. I always liked people watching, but it didn't amuse me today. Too nervous and emotional to get caught up on the silly things people do when they don't think anyone's watching. Maybe I'll go up now. Perhaps my room is ready early? Beats sitting down here waiting alone. I asked at the information desk where to go. I had packed away the pamphlets. Dummy. Deposited on the eleventh floor, I stood among the bank of elevators, confused. Which way? I followed a sign saying Neurology, and an arrow written on it, and found myself at a vast nursing station filled with charts, whiteboards and people.

"Where're you headed? You look lost?" A nurse behind the counter asked.

"I'm here for seizure monitoring?"

"Go down that hallway to the left to a blue-painted door. You can walk right in. Take care, hon."

Deep breath in, slow breath out. I turned to my destination, walking to meet my maker, my carry-on bag trudging behind me. I entered the unit, greeted by friendly faces behind a desk. It took up most of the space in the middle of the room, flanked by four rooms, two on each side. Right in front of the desk was a stationary bike. Glancing at it with raised eyebrows, I introduced myself. No sooner had my name left my lips, then a bell started ringing. The nurses sprung from their chairs and hurried to one room. Questions flew out of the mouth of the man who got there first. Where are you — what's your name—what day is it? Remember the word elephant and the colour pink. What's this? He held up a pen. The door closed and I couldn't hear any more. The person in the bed was staring off into space, not responding to the questions. Is that how I look? I wondered. I didn't know. No one has ever described what I'm like during my seizures other than eyes open, a blank expression, a vacant stare, and unresponsive. I stood looking at posters stuck to the wall at the entrance and the pamphlets mounted on the opposite wall.

"Linda? Hi. Sorry to leave you standing there. Let's get you settled." The nurse who'd responded to the alarm walked over to me and pointed to the room next to the patient who'd set off the alarms. He was slender, of average height, with black hair and brown eyes. He spoke with a slight accent I couldn't place. His calm demeanour had helped reduce my nervousness, and I'd felt myself relax a bit.

"That's ok. No worries." He'd directed me to my room, a windowless box with a glass sliding door, a cupboard, and some shelves. On one wall hung a computer screen and a keyboard tray suspended below, a chair in the other corner underneath a TV mounted above the door. The bed took up most of the room, leaving about a foot on either side — enough room for one to manoeuvre around.

"You can place your things in the cupboard. Please try to keep a clear pathway along the side of the bed in case we need to administer medication." Glancing over my clothes, he continued. "You can use a hospital gown or PJs or whatever. Make sure the top buttons up because once we put the electrodes on, you won't be able to pull anything over your head. You're best to change in the washroom here, as you're on video 24/7. The tech will be by once you're all settled to get you hooked up." He turned and then remembered something.

"Oh yeah, my name is Eric. I'm your nurse until tonight." He smiled and left.

I stood for a moment, not sure what to do. I might as well unpack and get changed. Not much else to do. My bag was jam-packed. The instructions were self-explanatory. Washroom? Oh yeah, right here outside my room. Convenient. When I stepped out of my cell, the woman sitting behind a screen at the desk piped up when she saw me.

"Oh, wait, you can't go in there." She pointed to a cord that ran under the bathroom door back to the room next to mine. "Someone's using it. See that? When you see a cord leading into the bathroom, that lets you know your neighbour is in there. You share this bathroom and those over there share the other one." I nodded and backed into my room to wait. It wasn't long before the door opened and an older man appeared. He had what looked like a stocking over his head with wires dangling down to a sling purse. The cord that ran along the floor hung from an opening in the pouch.

"It's all yours." Needing to pee. I didn't waste any time getting up and out. The bathroom wasn't large, but it's not like we would take any baths or showers. Closing the door behind me, I reached to lock it and found there wasn't one. Hmm, Okay. Interesting. Afraid the door would swing open at any moment, I changed, peed, and headed back to my room. A woman was in the corner by the computer, clicking away on the keyboard.

"Oh, great. You're back. I'm Opal, I'm one technologist who will look after you. If you're ready, we can go put your electrodes on and get you hooked up." She had a kind face, her eyes showing sympathy for what I was to go through. Leading the way, we twisted down hallways filled with discarded linen carts and chairs to a room. Opal waved me to the chair and began gathering cables, gauze, bottles and a stocking.

"This won't hurt, but the glue stinks like hell. So, I apologize in advance. Is this your first time on a seizure ward? You're from BC. Ever been to Alberta before?" She chattered away while working on my head, buzzing around like a bee looking for nectar.

"Yes, yes, and yes. I've been to Edmonton and Grande Prairie. It's my first time in Calgary."

I tried to sit still as she used a pen of some sort to mark my scalp, using a bit of pressure to make sure she would find them afterwards. Next came the jumble of colour coded wires attached to a little box the size of a Walkman. As she worked, I sat there wondering what's next. Oh man, she wasn't kidding. I wrinkled my nose as soon as she unscrewed the lid on the glue. My hypersensitive sense of smell, overwhelmed by the fumes, transported me back to when my brother worked on his model cars and balsam wood planes. It wreaked like model glue and contact cement. I could taste it in my mouth. Sensing my distaste, Opal promised,

"It's only bad when we're putting the electrodes on. The smell goes away after a while. The odour will disappear before you know it."

"I'm going to hold you to that. I have a sensitive nose and could be a drug dog; it's that keen." I could hear her chuckle as she finished up. Netting in place, she looped the pouch over one shoulder, letting it hang across in the front, and placed the little box inside.

"Okay, done. Let's get you back and connected." Back in the room, she attached the long telephone cable to my box and ran a diagnostic, asking me to open and close my eyes to get a baseline.

"We're all set. Need to test your button." She attached one final cord, a small cylinder with a red button resembling the ones used on Jeopardy at one end.

"Test." she bellowed.

"Thanks," Eric responded.

"Whenever you have a seizure, you need to press the button to 'mark' it. That will let us know to inspect the readings from the EEG. You're all set, Linda. Let me know if you have questions." Turning at the door, she had one last instruction. "Oh, and make sure you stay on camera at all times. We wouldn't want you to have a seizure without catching it on film." You could tell by her voice and the look in her eyes she was serious.

The room was narrow, lit by fluorescent tubes in need of replacement. I could hear soft voices outside the glass doors, but they did not mask the sounds of beeping machinery coming from other rooms similar to mine. It felt strange to be in a hospital, far removed from the familiar. The doctors and nurses were new to me, their faces a blur as I struggled to apply names to them. It didn't seem right that I must travel outside my province to seek the care I needed, and I tried to avoid that victim mentality one gets caught up in when faced with health issues. Never the type to succumb to a 'woe is me' mind set; I was stronger than that. Or so I had thought.

Left to my own defences, wrapped up in thoughts of what had been, the now, and what will be, was an inner turmoil foreign to my old self. The woman I had been. Positive, outgoing, always pushing to learn and grow. Not one to stagnate in the mire of doubt and uncertainty. That was then. Today, I'm withdrawn. My sleep patterns vary. Some nights I sleep well but wake exhausted; other times I wake early and can't calm my mind and doze off again. I've lost the reins and the control over my destiny. Lost in a world where my mind short circuits at will. A Tormentor from within attacks from the shadows, laying waste to my sanity, the heart of my being. I was here to repair the wiring in my scrambled brain. Cut out the loose connections, sending mixed messages, creating distortions spreading throughout my body. Ripples of motion like when a stone hits the smooth surface of a lake, sending a message to the shore, saying: I am here, you can not ignore me.

Sitting in my 9 x 9 cell, as I called it, must be what an inmate might feel surrounded by white walls and a door you can see through but limited in freedom of movement. I would think anyone having claustrophobic tendencies could feel the effects of walls and ceiling closing in. They warned me there wasn't a lot of space in the rooms and that was a fact! Very little airspace separated the bed from the walls on either side, and the distance to the door wasn't much more. A couple of drawers and a narrow cabinet were all the storage I had. They mounted the TV in the corner, high to avoid bumping one's noggin. Your basic hospital issue arm chair squeezed itself in the corner, reducing the footprint around the bed. The bed tray was a constant annoyance. It swung this way, over there, then here, as they took my blood pressure and checked electrodes. The added complication of my "leash" caught up and around the tray's wheels and post made manoeuvring a chore. Not all the rooms were equal. The two inside 'cabins' were of the same formation: a bed, cabinet and drawers, two shelves, a chair and TV. Two of the walls held the equipment for monitoring, and any emergencies. The 'outside' cabins were larger and had additional storage as a wide window ledge running the length of the room. Had more of a bedroom vibe compared to the shrouded darkness of a cave with lights as torches as mine had been. Regardless of the accommodations, the crew of nurses, doctors, and techs more than made up for the sparse surroundings and lack of activities.

As I got to know my cellmates, I proved to be a troublesome patient. I can still hear Opal's voice, "Linda. Get back on camera. If you insist on socializing, at least move further into the room, so you're within the camera's range." My 'leash' was long enough to take me across the unit. When my boredom got the best of me, I ventured out to chat.

They reduced my medication that night and again the next day, hoping to trigger a seizure. My morning routine composed of 8 am breakfast, the morning vitals check, and a makeshift sponge bath in the tiny bathroom, crosswords, reading and playing games on my iPad. The doctor would make his rounds with a full entourage of a nurse, technologist, and fellow. It was quite the procedure. Our closed doors allowed them to discuss each patient in private. They shuffled into a room, close the door, review the previous day's recordings, next steps and answer questions. Out they would come and close the door: next victim, next door. The severity of each case determined the time spent in each room. Labelled A, B, C, D. I was in D and the last one seen.

## **My Lifesaver arrives**

I felt like a speck in the room as they stood there surrounding my bed. It's surprising that four, sometimes five, people could fit. Dr. Young was intimidating to me the first few times. He seemed taller than he was and a presence about him that demanded respect. Short salt and pepper hair, black-rimmed glasses, and cropped sideburns and goatee. He was the epitome of what a doctor and professor would look like. It was pure luck, a fluke, how he became my epileptologist. He was standing in my doorway about to leave when he turned and asked,

"Who's your neurologist?" My blank stare prompted him to ask again. "Linda? Do you have a neurologist here?"

"No, I have Dr. Edwards back home in BC."

"I know that, but have you seen anyone here in Alberta?"

"No, I only have Dr. Edwards, no one else. " With brow furrowed and lips tightened together, he glanced at the corkboard mounted on the wall. It listed the meds I was on, tracked the removal of each, and my neurologist. Sighing, he turned to me and stated,

"I'm your neurologist." He smiled and left. Okay, then. I guess that's that.


They removed my meds as my brain wasn't cooperating. It went dormant, so to speak, and didn't want to come out and play. I'd been on antiseizure medication since March 2015, almost a year. I'd started on two, which were increased to four last August, and they still hadn't kept things under control. What was going to happen when they stopped giving them to me without the usual weaning process? I spent more time listening to music to distract myself and to keep from dwelling on the 'what if?' After lunch, I'm left alone to fill the hours as best as I can. Sometimes a doctor would return to grill me for more information. Their job was to be the detective to gather evidence to answer when the seizures occurred, when they'd started, etc.


It was Dr. Ivy who found me crying. Devon had informed me he was taking an anti-depressant. It wasn't so much the drug, but the fact he went to a walk-in clinic and saw a doctor who had no clue about his medical history. She said I needn't worry. The medication was a standard one for depression. It was hard being away from him. I felt helpless, useless. He was twenty-one, but still my baby. We only had each other, no one else. Alcohol killed his dad died when Dev was only twelve. If the antidepressant wasn't enough, he took out a loan and bought a car with his girlfriend. He never once asked for my advice or even hinted they were going to do this. I had been in the financial services industry for over thirty years. That was a bitter pill to choke down and took its toll on my mental state. I was alone and felt I'd failed him as a mother for not being there when I'd thought my son needed me. There I lay, attached to a 'leash.' Forced to share a bathroom with a stranger, eating hospital food and sponge bathing. It wasn't Club Med, I wasn't on holiday, and my brain still refused to fire off flares despite the doctors stripping away my meds.

## **Journal Entry February 12, 2016**

*Here I sit—hasn't been a week yet, and it feels like forever. I talk to Mom, Dev, text Margaret and my brother, Jim, update friends via text or messenger, daily. They'd made drastic cuts to my meds since the 8th. I was down to 50 mg each—2 x per day of the Dilantin and Lamotrigine. Not very much in the scheme of things and compared to what I was taking before. Sleep deprivation is one way to trigger a seizure and is the next step the doctors want to take to force my brain to cooperate.*

I was nervous. Part of me had wanted it to work, but deep down I'd hoped it wouldn't. To have gone through another seizure, as I'd had before, terrified me despite being in a safe and controlled setting. But I couldn't have stayed there forever, could I? My worries had been unfounded. I had had no seizures like on my sister's boat or back in March, just lots of solid waves. Countless times I pushed that jeopardy button as each wave hit. The odours were overpowering as they preceded the rushing sensations. Starting deep in my belly, they washed up and over my head. Even with none of the larger events, it had been a successful night. Between my worry about Dev and his mental state and lack of sleep—ten to eleven waves and nine odours recorded in less than a 24-hr period.

Dr. Young then ordered CT (Computed Tomography), MRI (Magnetic Resonance Imaging), PET (Positron Emission Tomography) and two SPECT (Single Photon Emission

Computed Tomography) scans as part of his investigation. The SPECT scan creates three-dimensional images of the brain on the computer. This allows neurologists to visualize the changes in blood flow when a seizure begins. Those with epilepsy often have changes in blood flow that are specific to areas of the brain when a seizure begins. By comparing scans before and during seizures, doctors can identify where a seizure originates.

For these, the technologist injected radioactive dye and then placed me in for scanning. Olivia, the technologist on duty that day, placed plastic on the floor of my room and sealed the gaps with tape to avoid contamination in the event of a spill. It was as if she were preparing for asbestos removal. Next, she'd brought in an IV pole with a bag of orange liquid that hung from the hook and attached it to my IV. It'd been quite the procedure, and I'd had to do it twice. When I felt a wave coming on, I was to press the button, and she would run in and release the dye into the IV. A few hours later, they would send me for my scan. I had seen them do this with another patient, and it had taken a few attempts before they achieved success. I'd nailed it on the first go. For the second one, they didn't want me to have any seizures. They needed to get a look at my brain while it was in neutral, not in full throttle. After a few attempts, we achieved the desired results.

**From:** Linda

**Sent:** February 14, 2016 3:05 PM

**To:** Margaret

**Subject:** Update

*Dr. Young came in this afternoon. Said the seizures have settled down with the new drug. He asked how I was doing, said I was emotional, felt flushed, felt kind of frozen/paralyzed but can move. Melanie, the nurse, asked if I had any sensations such as numbness or pins and needles...I said yes. Also feeling dopey as he had forewarned me. Asked me if I thought it was the drug, I said I think it's the entire package...has felt like a roller coaster ride. He will not increase the Topamax today, will see how it goes and will review again tomorrow. Still figures discharge on Tues after PET scan. He is going to have the neurosurgeon come see me on Tues before I leave to discuss the surgery process/details. If this happens, I'm going to give them your email address and to forward the info to you for any further questions. If that doesn't happen, then when I come back to see Dr. Young for follow up, he will try to coordinate the appointments for the same day. I can then bring questions you may have with me (or you come with me on that trip). I asked if he knew what the approx. Wait times were for surgery he said a matter of months. So, I'm putting it in my head that it won't be until the end of the year, at the earliest, no reason, just cause. If I understood him, Dr. Young will continue as my neurologist here in Calgary and I'm assuming I will continue with Dr. Edwards in BC.*

*I think that's it for now. Lol.*

*Love to ya both,*

Xoxoxox

Linda




Dr. Young proved to be another Dr. Terry, a hard shell on the outside with a soft centre hidden from view. With his dedication to his profession, research, and teaching, I considered myself fortunate to have him as my doctor. I could feel the empathy in his voice as he stood next to my bed, explaining the test results and the next steps. I sat like a meek schoolgirl listening to the teacher. *Good news. I'm a candidate for a temporal lobe resection. A what?*

"Dr. Taylor will explain the procedure to you. Based on what we've seen, we estimate a 70% chance of reducing your seizures by as much as 50% — even becoming seizure free. You would be on some form of medication ongoing, but you'll see an improvement in your quality of life. You might drive again and return to work. Our prognosis is very positive."

Stunned, I sat there, nodding, trying to take in everything. I jotted down cryptic notes, trying hard not to miss a word he'd said. "We need memory tests completed to create a baseline of your cognitive functions before surgery. Then we repeat them a year later to see if there are any changes. Will you be staying in Alberta for a bit? We can put a rush on it so you can do them before you head home."

"I can stay at my brother's in Leduc if I have to?"

"Good." With a tap on my table tray, he smiled and left.

*Wow. Surgery. Wow.* The reality of it hit me like a five-ton baby elephant. Yes, the whole point of coming here was to see if I was eligible for surgery. That had been an *'if'* now it's a *'when.' Jeez, Louise. Wow.* The rest of the day I spent staring around my room, letting the news trickle through my neurons to the messaging centre, hoping to make sense of it all.

Dr. Taylor sat with me on the day they'd discharged me. Perched on a chair too short for his 6-foot frame, he spoke of the usual risks and the possibility I could lose some of my vision—the upper left. It may be temporary or permanent. They would cut the side of my head open at the temporal lobe, peel the skin back to slice through the bone and cut out the scar. Then the bone glued together, the skull plate set in place and stapled shut. I signed the consent form, giving him the green light to mess with my head. Go in, look at every nook and cranny. Remove a part of me that operates my body—allows me to think and feel. The thought of it all was staggering. That I was here on my own, making a decision that could affect my life, was daunting. No one could understand or appreciate what I was going through. No one could unless they were going through it or been through it themselves. After he left, I floated in another dimension, the past weeks replaying like a movie— one frame at a time but not in sequence. The pictures were all jumbled. After a few moments, they sped up, moving so fast they became a cloudy vision—one melting into another, spinning so fast I thought I would take flight.

*[The brain is a complex organ divided into sections, each one responsible for various functions and body parts. The Temporal Lobe is home to memories of the past, present, and future. If it isn't 'packed' right, it alters how well one can access the contents, pull them in and out at will to share. If not replaced in the correct order, they get jammed, making it difficult to reach—to find them.]*

They scheduled my memory tests for the end of February. My brother Jim arranged for us to stay with our childhood friends Chris and Jerry to avoid the two-hour drive each way from Leduc. It was so lovely of them to take us in. We picked up our friendship where it left off thirty years ago, as if no time had passed.

We arrived early at Foothills Hospital the next morning for the memory testing.

"So, tell me, Linda, what has changed for you since your diagnosis?" Laura asked. She was the head of the neuropsychology department, and we sat with her before the examinations. Laura moved her chair closer to give me her undivided attention. Laura was young, looked to be in her thirties, with rich mahogany brown hair. It hung just above her shoulders, not touching the grey tweed suit jacket she wore. Her ivory skin glowed and her emerald-green eyes stood out against the backdrop of her wavy hair. Her smile was inviting, and her posture relaxed and welcoming. The other lady was my examiner, Madeline. Maddy, which she preferred, leaned against the desk, observing. Dressed in casual slacks, a white buttoned blouse and pale blue cardigan, she resembled that of a high school teacher being introduced to her newest student.

"Well, I can't drive, can't work, can't travel alone. My entire life has turned upside down and sideways. I've lost my independence." My words caught in my chest, blocked by a massive lump, making speech difficult. Jim sat beside me, listening. It was essential to have a friend or a family member present to provide an outside perspective.

"Linda has always been fiercely independent. She had to. Linda raised her son on her own and managed her finances well. It's been tough on her, but she's strong and determined. It's how she's gotten this far." Jim said.

"I bet it has—such a life-altering illness. So, Linda, we will conduct some tests over the next couple of days. I will submit the compiled report of results to your epileptologist, surgeon, and GP back home. Would you also like a copy of it?"

"Yes, please. That would be great."

"Okay, Linda, all done." She rose, and we followed suit, shook hands and left; passed the waiting area that would become Jim's reading nook during my testing. Jim walked me to the elevators. My eyes had become misty, and with my diminished sense of direction, had made it easy to get lost.

We returned the next day, and Jim made himself comfortable in his reading nook. Maddy greeted us at the reception and led me back down the same corridor as yesterday to her office. It was a cramped space filled with overstuffed cabinets, piles of books and papers scattered everywhere. There was enough room for two, no more. We sat at a table along a wall and across from her desk. We sat angled towards each other. There wasn't the room to sit perpendicular to the table, to face each other. Maddy started my examination by flipping cards imprinted with different images and asked me to name them. Simple items such as flower, house, car, tree. Once we'd run through those, she set them aside and grabbed another stack. This pile had geometric shapes and, again, Maddy flipped through them, giving me a moment to study each. She then instructed me to draw any of the shapes I could recall. She hadn't expected me to produce a Renoir or Picasso.

"Just do the best you can. Your artistic ability isn't what's being tested." Maddy said with a smile. It had relieved me since the best I could draw was stickmen, and even those were sketchy. We ran through these twice before we'd moved to the desk, and she pulled out what I'd called a puzzle board. It was a cardboard square with multiple boxes cut out with removable pieces. Some had red dots, others were black, the rest were all white. I was to replicate a diagram by placing the part in the correct position on the board—an adult version of a baby's first jigsaw puzzle. Next, Maddy read brief sentences from a card, and asked me to repeat them back. To add to the challenge, she read a short story and asked specific questions, such as what is the name of the man in the story? Was he doing anything? Was he sleeping? Or eating? Was it raining? Or snowing? What was he experiencing? Was he angry? Did he have a problem at work? Etc. etc. She even tested my hearing. The concentration and mental acuity I'd needed to recall the information drained my energy, making me weary. I could feel the pressure inside my head as I'd pushed it to work. The force I placed upon it wouldn't have been any different from the effort of lifting weights. The difficulty in recalling simple, essential words and pictures was a surprise to me. I prided myself on my excellent memory; this test showed me just how much I'd lost. I was exhausted. I blamed the meds and prayed that was the reason for the deterioration. The tests were now behind me. I said goodbye to Foothills, knowing I'd be back in a few months.

Jim and I spent the drive back to Leduc chattering as we used to in the old days, comfortable in each other's company. We'd re-established the bond we had in our youth — strengthening the cords that weaved it together. It felt good being with my brother again.

Two days later, it was time to head home. To my space and bed. To my son, and to sit and wait. Surgery could be as early as April or May, and I wouldn't speak with Dr. Young until June over the phone. But my brain had other plans. My next seizure occurred two months after returning home and was the most embarrassing one yet.

*[I was a firm believer that your choices in life could come back and smack you in the face like a boomerang, causing you to re-evaluate the past. Those deeds of long ago determined how kind fate would be and whether karma was a friend or foe.]*

The mere thought of surgery was terrifying. It was like facing the end of time and a blank existence. Dr. Young adjusted the meds to help me through the weeks until my return. To chain the evil and suppress its onslaught. It worked for a while, but the power was too great and the links that bound it were too fragile.

## **Back Home—Now we wait**

## **Journal Entry March 2, 2016**

*I got home on February 26th. Walking through the door into the hallway taking in the cheery yellow painted walls and the warmth radiating from the brown and grey laminate floors blanketed me in comfort. I had flopped onto the couch, a sense of gratitude filling my heart. But it felt weird as I was away for so long. I'd been away for just as long as I'd had back in August 2015 at Sullivan District, but I hadn't been near my friends and Mom, Margaret and Devon. And now I had to go back. How did I feel? Calmer than before; maybe. a lot of progress made since August. Saw the neurosurgeon before I left the unit and signed the consent forms. Now all I had to do was wait... again.*

*Up till then, I'd only had one wave (just the other day) and no odours. Thus, the new med and dosages seemed to have things under control. The Topamax dosage was still increasing, so would reduce the chances of any further activity even more. Surgery? Yeah, as the reality of it seeped into my conscious, my gut said, 'back away.' A nervous energy had begun to boil, swirling around my stomach rising to choke the oxygen from reaching my lungs. It wasn't just the thought of someone cutting into my skull—taking a piece of bone out and the scar on my brain–then putting it back together—YUCK. It was the afterwards that frightened me. No matter how many tests they did, no one could predict the outcome until after it's all said and done. My memory may not improve (or it could worsen) my mood/personality could change or, if I'm not wired as most people, it could affect my speech. Even my vision, too. And what about my disability coverage should my vision become impaired? They won't cover me for blindness, but is that just for natural causes?*

*I knew I shouldn't have thought about all those "what ifs," but it was difficult not to. I spent a lot of time during those days convincing myself that everything'd be okay. That I just had to deal with one day at a time. To just take one day at a time.*

# Chapter Seven

## **April 2016—Waiting Again**

I tried to keep my mind off the surgery. The thoughts of a knife splicing through bone, tissue, nerves, and muscle were unbearable. But I couldn't stop them. Even in my dreams, they'd continued. I'd dreamt of the surgeon cutting through my scalp before the anaesthetic had kicked in, and they couldn't hear my screams because of the oxygen mask. My arms were strapped down and I couldn't lift them to remove it. Or I'd dreamt I'd gotten through the surgery and wasn't able to recognize anyone after and couldn't see out of my left eye. While Mom and I prepared for our trip back to Alberta in May, an application to WestJet for their One Person One Fare program was submitted and approved. It'd allowed me to travel with a companion at half the cost, a buy one, get one deal. My companion had to be over eighteen and capable of looking after me. The only cost for them was the applicable taxes for their ticket.

My seizure activity hadn't stopped—the waves and putrid odour continued despite the adjustments to my meds. But that hadn't stopped me from venturing out, only slowed my progress. When it'd hit, it forced me to grab hold of the closest post, bench, or what have you, to steady myself. The rush of feeling, the sensation of a tide hitting the rocks was so strong it could've knocked me down. An odour often preceded the wave—that same unpleasant scent I'd had on the boat. For me, with a delicate nose susceptible to the faintest whiff, this had been almost worse than the waves. It'd been during a trip to Home Depot that such an event occurred. The store is along a busy avenue, nestled among condos, shops, and offices. A half hour's walk from home, crossing major roadways and across an overpass suspended above the freeway. The steady stream of traffic on my left headed in both directions combined with the loud Peterbilt's, pickups, and cars racing underneath me created a whirlwind inside my head. The fast movements, honking horns, the roar of engines wreaked havoc upon my heightened senses. It'd become a personal challenge to make the trek across without feeling panicked - heart racing - breaking out in a sweat - wanting to curl into a ball kind of panic.

In the back corner where the metal racking along two sides meet, I found the object of my quest: seven feet up and too high to reach. Back then, it'd never occurred to me to order anything online except for my groceries. I'd had two feet and could walk. What I couldn't carry home would come back with me in a cab or on the bus. I knew exactly what I wanted. Brown wicker side tables to go with the club chairs out on my deck. With or without glass hadn't mattered, only colour and size. Way up on the top shelf, I spied exactly what I was looking for. I'd just needed help to get them down. As I turned to find a store associate, I felt it. A surging tide from my core that'd lifted up and over me. A G-force sensation that was twenty times worse than the fastest rollercoaster, causing me to stumble into the rack beside me. While I waited it out, the putrid smell surpassed the receding rush and filled my nostrils to overflowing, to where I tasted it.

I grabbed the cold steel and breathed through it as best I could, but it didn't help. The urge to run was immense, but would've solved nothing. I recall pulling out my phone to call... someone. I don't remember who or why. I stared at it and then dropped my arm. There was no point trying to call anyone. My phone was useless. With all the concrete and metal around me, the signal couldn't reach outside to connect. *I should go sit,* I told myself and turned to move around the tower of metal to the furniture displays. Intuition had told me standing was not a good idea.

I woke in the emergency, my head heavy from the Ativan pumped into my system and the explosion that erupted inside my brain. Confused, sleepy, weak, and beat up, it took hours before I'd returned to my normal self—my baseline.

I was told I'd had a seizure in the Home Depot. That someone had found me sitting on some patio furniture. No one knew how long it had lasted, or how much time had passed before someone noticed me and called 911.

*[Ativan (Lorazepam) is used to treat all types of seizures, with its rapid absorption into the system it is often used as rescue medication for prolonged seizures.]*

*[It's taken a long time before I could recall the events leading up to the seizure. To this day, what had happened when I'd turned to sit down remains a blank. I vaguely recall entering a note on my phone and then turning. But the rest is dark, like a shutter on a camera closing, blocking the image before it, and no longer visible to the one behind the lens.]*

Margaret brought me fresh clothes so I could go home. It'd seemed odd that it was necessary. *'Where were my pants, shirt, and bra? I know I wasn't naked and my outing not a dream. So, where were they?'* Only my pants, socks, and shoes survived, and yet, I couldn't wear the pants? While I'd sat seizing on the furniture, my bladder relaxed and spilled its contents over me, the pants, and the cushion. Just as a toddler in potty training would. When I heard what'd happened, I almost fainted. The horror and embarrassment overwhelmed me. I was mortified, disgusted, ashamed.

*[When the paramedics arrive and I'm unconscious, there's no regard for clothing or modesty. Shirts, jackets, and underclothes are cut away to make room for stickers and wires attached to a portable ECG. It is imperative to determine the status of my heart to rule out an attack. Over the years, I've lost count of how many articles of clothing I've had to replace as the EMT's worked on my body.]*

It took weeks before I could joke about it, commenting on how the staff had a Wanted Picture of me in their lunchroom, how it was no longer a viable option to meet guys with my single friends. "Find yourself a new wingman," I'd laughed.

To this day, that seizure has been the most embarrassing one I've ever experienced.

*[Losing awareness and not knowing what transpired in that block of time was freaky, an-out-of-this-life experience. The best way to describe it would be: Falling asleep suddenly with no warning while carrying on with normal everyday things; a swimmer fighting to reach the surface, not knowing his struggle to break free - of the dominant force dragging him down; to come to in strange surroundings, confused, beat up, weak and with no memory of how you got there. It's like you died and came back. One moment you are alive - the next darkness and a foggy veil of confusion and disbelief. A child waking from a nightmare, not sure of what scared him - screaming in terror.]*

*\*\*Journal Entry May 8, 2016\*\**

*Things have moved along since my most recent seizure. After Margaret faxed over the consultation notes from emergency to Dr. Young, my follow up moved up to April 27th.*

Margaret had me prepare a list of questions to ask, which I'd emailed to her.

**From:** *Linda*

**Sent:** *April 26, 2016 3:30 PM*

**To:** *Margaret*

**Subject:** *Questions for tomorrow's call*

*Hey, here's what I've come up with so far for the call with Dr. Young tomorrow.*

*1. Pros and Cons - worse case scenario - moods - behaviour     - memory issues*

*2. How long in hospital after surgery?*

*3. How long would need to stay in Calgary after surgery?*

*4. Rehabilitation Process?  - here or in Calgary?*

*- if here, will he refer back to Edwards or will I deal with GP?*

*5. Medication - continue with current prescriptions? - for how long? - who do I see/talk to about changes?*

*6. Follow-up Process—here or in Calgary?*

*- if here, will he refer back to Edwards or will I deal with GP?*

*7. Recovery Time?*

*And depending on worse case scenario, that surgery is not an option - What's the next step? Also, would like to get copies of all test results, etc. for my records.*

*Anything you can think of to ask?*

*Linda*

It had been a relief to have had Margaret there for the call. She'd made notes and emailed them to me, Mom, and Jim.

**From:** *Margaret*
**Sent:** *May 2, 2016 7:17 AM*
**To:** *Mom; Jim; Linda.*
**Subject:** *Summary of T-con with neurologist*

*We had a t-con with Dr Young last Wednesday · All the testing confirmed that all Linda's seizures come from the temporal lobe on the RIGHT side of her brain.*

*· Her verbal memory testing was all normal*

*· She is an ideal surgical candidate with at least a 70% chance of being seizure free.*

*Current medical therapy has only a 3-4% chance of being seizure free (and given recent events, I would hazard to say it is less than that—my words)*

*· Linda is right handed—this means her verbal memory and language skills are housed in the LEFT side of her brain. The area of scarring is on the RIGHT, and so surgery won't affect language and memory. She should not have chronic memory loss.*

*· The current behavioural/processing/memory issues are likely related to her medications, and he anticipated will improve once the meds are weaned off.*

*· No need to see surgeon pre-op. Usual risks—infection, anesthetic, etc. were touched on by Dr. Taylor (the surgeon) when he saw Linda in Calgary just before discharge.*

*· Dr. Young said to anticipate a 4-5 day hospital stay.*

*· Will need to be in Calgary several weeks post-op. (and I think he meant Alberta–so going to Jim's should be fine but need to confirm)*

*· Driving is fine–but there seems to be some inconsistency re when she can fly. MOA at Taylor's office wasn't sure and Dr Young suggested no flying for "some weeks" but no one has been specific*

*· She will feel tired in first 3 months "brain takes lots of energy to heal"*

*Follow up appts · Neurology–Dr. Young–needs to see at 3, 6 and 12 months post-op. · Surgeon–6-8 weeks post–op. I asked MOA about combining that appt with 3 month neuro follow up–one a bit early and one a bit late, and she felt this was doable. · She does need to connect with Dr. Edwards post-op and have local neuro follow up with him. He is aware. · No meds will be weaned for the first year, with exception of the Clobazam. So still some unknowns,.... But this is all we know for now.*

*Margaret*

The next step had been a call from the surgeon's office with a date. Well, they hadn't messed around and I'd received the call the next day; they set the surgery for May 20th... It'd blown me away at how quickly they'd called. I hadn't expected it. I'd thought it wouldn't be for a week or two at least. If it wasn't for the Clobazam, it would've freaked me out—but I seemed calm about it. Even twelve days before we had to go, I'd still felt calm, untroubled, almost serene—It was difficult to put into words. Unemotional? Spock-like? Maybe? I still got overwhelmed with stuff and had problems comprehending certain things. But I also had moments where the clouds lifted and I'd feel "normal." Like my old self—almost. I was cold all the time—not the 'old me' at all. I knew I'd had to get back to life and not allow it to beat me—I had to take control. But it was hard. I occasionally went shopping with Mom and Dev or went on outings with friends, and it'd been okay. I told myself if I took it slow, I'd be fine. I'd been back up to four meds and had been taking them for three weeks, which had kept things under control as it had before. When I had my April seizure, I didn't have my medic alert bracelet on—it was broken and without it, it delayed the proper medical treatment I'd needed. Soon after my discharge, Mom had escorted me to the jeweller's and purchased a silver medic alert necklace. I've not taken it off since. Everything had fallen into place until the phone rang.

"Hi Linda, it's Karen. Are you in Calgary now?"

"No, we're set to leave in a few days."

"Well, I'm sorry, but we're having to postpone your surgery. An urgent case has come up, and we're unable to proceed. I'll be in touch once I've got a new date for you. So sorry for the inconvenience." My billowing sail lost its wind. No longer flapping, it'd hung from the rigging as if dangling from the end of a noose. All the preparations had been made, the airline tickets bought, and the hotel booked. I'd had mentally geared myself up for the most prominent major event in my life. And it'd been for nothing. I cried angry, defeated tears. *How could they do this to me?* My family consoled me as best as they could've. I got past it and had hit the reset button and moved forward and life had carried on. As days and weeks passed, the waiting had almost killed me. To have had the plug pulled so close to 'go time,' sent me swirling down the drain. No one but my journal knew to what degree it had played on my psyche.

*\*\*Journal entry—June 19, 2016\*\**

*I had a meltdown yesterday. It started after I checked the Canadian drug shortage list to see if any more of my drugs were listed. Margaret told me Fri that my Clobazam wasn't available anymore and to check with the pharmacy to see if they had any left. I have 55 pills left. I take 2 a day. The pharmacist said they had none. No one did. Will need to change my prescription – call your doctor. Lamotrigine is too.*

*I left Michelle another garbled message at Dr. Young's office regarding Clobazam. I won't have enough to cover me until my surgery in August.*

*I fell apart yesterday; I was shaking and couldn't stop crying. I called Margaret. She had me take an Ativan to help calm down. I packed a few things and they picked me up and brought me to Mom's. I stayed the night. I spend so much time alone. I'm afraid to go out by myself. I feel stupid for feeling that way, but I do. All my friends are busy. They try, but they have their own lives. We're coming into summer. People are taking off on vacations, working in their yards, heading off to BBQs.*

*Usually, being alone wouldn't be an issue. I was doing better before the last seizure. I was getting out for walks pretty much every day. Going further and further. I was getting stronger–toning. I am feeling a bit better about myself despite my situation. Then, as per usual, BAM, I'm kicked to curb again. A seizure happens. Out of the blue. This time, if it had happened about 15 min sooner, I'd be out walking and crossing the street. Now here I sit at my Mom's–feeling like a little girl again who can't look after herself. I know my frame of mind has not been reasonable. I've dug a hole and crawled into it, not even crying out for help much. I haven't been reaching out to friends. I get up- I eat–get dressed- play games and go on FB- do laundry when needed- pretend to cook (sometimes) and watch Netflix. Oh, and I nap and sleep.*

*I go out sometimes when I can get Dev to get motivated to take me. Otherwise, I'm at home. I haven't even been writing in here much — last entry- a month ago. I haven't also been listening to music. I can't remember the last time I put the stereo on. I haven't been reading either. As much as I want my independence, it's best that I stay with Mom for a while. Just for my emotional stability and to keep my sanity in line.*

# Chapter Eight

## **July 14, 2016–Paralysis**

The stress of waiting came to a head a week before Mom and I were to depart to Calgary. I'd been visiting my mom when another event hit. But it was different that time. I never lost consciousness and was aware of what my body was doing. It was frightening, as much for me as it was for her. She'd never seen a seizure before and hadn't any idea of what to do. It'd begun like the others, with an odour and a wave. My left arm couldn't move and my leg froze. The force within my head was like nothing I'd ever experienced. Rolling waves of pain and pressure exploded, creating a tidal wave that'd knocked my brain about. My neck stretched to the side, the veins and nerves still—muscle tissue stretched beyond endurance. Ativan hadn't helped. Feeling helpless, Mom called the paramedics. Shot up with drugs and removed to the emergency room, they'd placed me in a chair in a hallway; no beds available.

My nurse, older than most, had been unsympathetic, almost rude. She thought I had faked it, when my lifeless left arm hadn't lifted and I couldn't turn my head so she could blind me with her pin light. The wrinkles around her steel-blue eyes and at the corners of her thin lips had puckered and creased with displeasure. She spoke with clipped, stiff words, berating me as if I'd been a child. But Mom wouldn't allow it and like a protective mother bear, she raised her voice and with cold eyes glared at her,

"She can't move. Understand? She isn't able to lift her arm or leg. She can't even walk."

Faced with Mom's rage, she'd backed down. She stood as if to go, but then had turned and squatted in front of me. She then checked my temperature, had taken my pulse, and shone her penlight into my pupils. Her tasks completed, she'd stood and strode away. I can't remember if we ever saw a doctor and if we had, I've no idea what they said. A walker appeared. They wouldn't allow me to leave until I could stand and walked, using it for support. I spent hours signalling to my limbs to move, straining to send the messages from my head to ligaments, muscle and bone to stir. To restore the energy necessary to leave. But I hadn't any and they'd wanted me to stand up and walk out? Minutes passed before I'd gotten the courage to get up. With fingers clenched around the bar, I'd schooched to the edge of the seat, taken a deep breath, braced my arms, and stood up. My legs shook and pins and needles coursed up and down, awakening the nerves. It'd taken a bit, but I'd shuffled forward and could sit on the chair, stand up, and go again. Discharged, we'd headed back to Mom's.

By morning, I'd regained full capacity of my limbs. To move them took effort. They were limp, almost lifeless. Muscles, once strong, had become tired and heavy as if I'd just run a marathon. My trainer would've liked it if that had been the case. I'd even tried to count it as a workout. I'd figured that a seizure, like that one, should count as one or two sessions. My heart rate had been elevated - arm and leg muscles contracted - it'd last for over thirty minutes. A solid cardio workout in my books. My trainer hadn't agreed. But I knew what my body had gone through, and it hadn't been fun. I preferred my old seizures, the ones where I'd lose consciousness, unaware of what's going on. More dangerous, maybe, if out alone. But at least I wouldn't feel the lightning strikes and rolling thunder that'd had tormented my brain.

# Chapter Nine

*\*\*August 2016—Foothills Medical Centre,*

*Calgary—The Surgery\*\**

I laid on a stretcher waiting for transport to the MRI. I felt calmer than the day before because I was at the point of no return. The thought of my head spliced open was still daunting, and my heart pounded, echoing throughout my chest, sounding hollow. Other than my morning pills, my stomach was empty, amplifying the beats as they bounced off the lining.

Margaret stood next to the bed, patted my hand and said, "It's going to be okay. All they're doing is checking out the marbles in your head. They need to pull them out to find the bad marble. The trick is to make sure they don't mix them up and put the bad one back in. If they do, it will make you all wonky donkey."

Bursting out laughing, I told her she was a nut bar. A minute later, a porter wheeled me away. They took me down corridors to a waiting area in an alcove off to the side of a massive reception desk. I'd lain there listening to the hustle and bustle of nurses and doctors prepping for surgery. It felt like I was in a corral—beds lined up row upon row, like cattle waiting for the slaughter. I'd had no sense of the time passing as the minutes clicked by. People watching hadn't provided the amusement it usually did. There wasn't the steady flow of traffic passing by to have held my attention. I closed my eyes to escape the boredom and isolation—the loneliness. I'd almost drifted off when a gentle hand had touched my shoulder.

"Linda? I'm going to review your MRI and come back for a quick chat." I nodded my head, and watched as Dr. Taylor strode to the desk, his tall frame looming above everyone else. I listened to the exchange with the nursing staff about how well his weekend had been, their laughter and jokes. Returning to my stall, he'd sat down and ran through the procedure we'd talked about six months prior.

"So? Are you ready for this, Linda? How are you doing?" His voice was soft, his demeanour relaxed and calming.

"I'm doing great." And I was. Relaxed, all tension gone, taking in deep breaths, exhaling the stale warm air diffused any nervousness, keeping me calm and unconcerned — almost blasé.

"Okay, we're going to set up the OR, and then we're ready to go. I'll see you in there."

He then walked through the sliding doors. They looked and sounded like the ones you'd see on Star Trek, a hidden sensor that'd picked up your body's movement and opens just before you'd walk into them. I hadn't waited long before they wheeled me away. A quick bathroom stop, to avoid any accidents on the table and then I strolled into the room. It was full of people and machines and lights. Everyone bustled about as they set up the table, chattering away, oblivious of my presence. They had music playing, and the room had been cold. I assumed that they kept the temperature low, so they'd stay alert during the lengthy surgery. Good. I didn't want Dr. Taylor to fall asleep as he tinkered with my brain. The one thing about operating tables that always puzzled me, was how narrow they were. I'm definitely not what you'd call thin or chunky; I'm fat and often wondered if there'd ever been a patient who fell off the table as the anaesthesia took hold. After I'd settled onto the table, and covered with a warm blanket, they'd inserted the IV. They strapped my arms to my sides and then locked my head into position. I wasn't rolling off *anything*. With the sedative flowing into my veins, and a mask placed over nose and mouth,

I'd counted. Breathe in- one -two; breathe out - three - four and breathe-e-e a-n-d… gone.

**Post-Op—It's done**

The surgery had gone well, but my head disagreed. The throbbing pain overwhelmed my senses, was worse than any headache or strike to the noggin I'd ever experienced. The thump-thump-jab filled me beyond capacity. At that moment, if I could've hit rewind and changed my mind, I would have. The Tylenol every four hours couldn't break through to reach the epicentre of the torture. The Percocet administered through IV, had left me drugged up to where I wasn't eating or drinking. In and out of awareness, I barely touched the food trays they'd insisted on bringing. But even with the painkiller, I'd remained in agony. The nurses couldn't keep up with my requests for ice packs. I'd lain on my left side with the right side of the head covered in coolness, deadening the pain for brief moments. Margaret eventually cut off the Percocet. She'd said I had to be coherent enough to sit up and drink ice chips and slurp soup. My oxygen levels had dropped because of the lack of fluids entering my body. Between Margaret and the nurses, they forced me bit by painful bit from my prone state and forced me to leave my sanctuary. Doctors Taylor and Young enforced what they'd been telling me, and I'd had no choice but to get up and move. They'd explained that laying down all the time would cause pressure on the brain and push against the swollen tissue. I'd complied. I'd started to eat and drink and hobble the twenty steps to the bathroom and back. After five days, I was declared fit enough to leave my cocoon.

Discharged, Mom, Margaret and I headed back to our hotel room to await my brother. Mom and I had stayed in Leduc with my brother, Jim and his wife Carol for two weeks before we'd flown back home. Margaret had left earlier for Victoria to meet up with her husband, Barry, who awaited her return on their boat. They'd had plans to sail along the British Columbian coastline. I settled at Jim's with pain killers and Ativan at my bedside. The thumping in my head had reduced to the roar of a digger scraping rocks but hadn't disappeared. We spent our time reading, playing cards, and movies on Netflix. A day or two or three went by, one melted into another, no clear division between them.

**And the waves roll on Leduc, Alberta**

My waves; that sensation of water that washed over me, rushing up and encompassing my upper torso and head and then receding as if in retreat, was still there, but this time, I had pain.

The operation had altered the waves. They now pulled me up and hurtling me at the rocks and slammed me down over and over, beating the breath from me. They had never caused such discomfort before. Had always rushed to the head, then trickled over the edge. That day they'd held the full force of pressure, bursting through the defences I'd built to hold it back. On and on it'd gone. When it hadn't stopped, Mom called 911. Leduc Hospital doesn't have a neurological ward, so they transported me to Edmonton. Forty-five minutes I'd bounced in the back of the ambulance as they'd raced along the highway and city streets. We came to a halt at the emergency entrance to a queue of six ambulances. The University of Edmonton hospital is extremely busy and the wait times are long. The EMTs stayed with us until they moved me to a bed in the emergency room. They're required to stay and monitor their charge until released to the care of the emergency room nurses and doctors. It wasn't until afterwards I'd felt guilty. I had held up an ambulance and two medics outside of their jurisdiction. Tests completed, and they released me to my family's care. It had been a relief to be told that the seizure had caused no damage but next time take an Ativan.

Oh. Yeah. Nobody had mentioned that. *Duh.*

# Chapter Ten

## **Post Surgery—August 20, 2016—Back in BC**

Mom pulled rank and insisted I stayed with her until I could manage on my own. Dev was at school and worked part time, I really shouldn't be alone. I gave in to her request because if I'd been honest with myself, the thought of spending so many hours on my own had made me nervous. My energy levels had depleted and the brief flares of activity, were a constant reminder they hadn't left and still lurked in the background.

We hadn't taken long before Mom and I had settled into a morning routine. Most days I was awake first and had the coffee made, the cereal bowls, spoons and mugs out on the counter ready for the fruit, yogurt and granola. I left after a week; it was time to go. I had to move on and rebuild a new normal.

"Are you sure you're going to be alright? Dev isn't around during the day. Will you be ok?" The concern on Mom's face had been sincere—fear and love mingled in her voice—shone through her eyes.

"Mom. I'll be fine. I need to go home at some point and move around more. The stairs will be good for me. I need the exercise. I'll be fine." Poking at my jelly-belly, it was time I'd stopped lazing about. My muscle mass may have disappeared, but the rolls that expanded my midsection had multiplied. She didn't look convinced, but had known I would go. She hugged me hard and kissed my head, turning away before I could see the tears. That first night was paradise. Instead of the waves crashing into me, they'd lifted me up, carried me off, and lulled me into a peaceful slumber. You never know how much you miss your bed until you're forced to be somewhere else.

It felt great to be home again. Despite its comfort and the support of family and friends, the symptoms from prior to the operation had persisted. Waves continued and then increased as each month passed. The rising sensations now as much a part of me as breathing. The only difference had been the intensity. My waves were not the gentle lapping of water caressing the sand like before, but were strong rapids rushing over rocks, eroding all that stood in the way. I'd not only felt the pounding of those sensations, but the shrieking and writhing nerves the surgeon's saw had severed. The incision site was raw and washing my hair took time. Only the fingertips could rest on my scalp. Their touch could barely stroke the hair that'd grown back just above the bruised skin they clung to.

Nights were filled with dreams of the past; old acquaintances, co-workers, and childhood friends. The stories were illogical: men and women, dead and alive, long forgotten as I moved from job to job, city to city. They made no sense, were not plausible. Characters from different aspects of my life, from various points in time, paired together in the oddest situations. And to this day, they've continued to disturb my sleep.

Remembering things was difficult. I'd write notes for everything. Tracked my waves, the seizures, any Ativan I'd taken, and logged anything out of the ordinary: every little twinge, prickle, emotion, sleep disturbance, other such oddities. My conversations, to do lists, questions, and worries, medication changes and missed dosages added to the ever-growing journal of symptoms and weirdness. I'd become obsessed, which had zapped my energy. I'd been so in tuned with every nuance of my body, which had overworked my fragile mind, that on countless occasions I'd left the house just to turn back at the corner and check that I'd taken my meds. My detailed entries documented the boring facts of my existence and had shown me just how much those early days had affected me. My struggle to understand what'd happened, and an intense need to regain control of my life and body, and how traumatic it'd been. And still is.

*September 8, 2016: The Healing Starts*

We began the weaning process of my anti-seizure medication a month after surgery. It may have been too early, but the amount of medication I'd been on was excessive. Dr. Edwards wanted to see how my brain would react to being on one less drug and I agreed with some hesitation. The dosage had dropped by only one quarter before my waves returned, increasing in frequency as the weeks went by.

By September 28, 2016, my doctors said stop. It had been too soon after surgery to consider reducing my meds any further, and I continued on with the current mix of meds.

During those early days, I'd known deep down that the operation had failed. I would spend most days curled up on the couch or bed and suffer in silence, depressed. The continuance of my wave activity was disheartening, and I withdrew further, becoming a recluse. I was like a ghost wandering the days, mourning the loss of my earthly body. All I could focus on was myself and what I'd lost. I argued with family and friends when they offered advice to pull me out of the crevice I'd wedged myself into. My outlook on life held little hope of a future beyond the day-to-day hell I found myself in. My positive outlook had diminished to where it no longer existed.

When I tried putting my feelings into words to my family and friends, they couldn't understand. 'Find a hobby.' 'Go for a walk and get some fresh air.' 'Don't sweat the small stuff.' These were the responses I got. 'What do you know about it?' 'You've got no clue!' 'Never mind! You just don't get it!' were my come backs. My frustration and anger so great, my insides shook—a tightly wound coil about to spring—letting loose all the emotions I tried to bury. I developed a short fuse ignited by the slightest spark. My thoughts and feelings written in my journal had stirred so many negative emotions, which alarmed me. Not only did I feel depressed, but my body did too. It felt as though a weight pulled me down, pushed the air out and made it hard to breathe. Worried about my negative state of mind, I brought it up with Dr. Edwards.

"That's a common occurrence after temporal lobe surgery and a side effect of most of your meds. I'll prescribe Citalopram in a small dose to start. And I'll place a referral into the Mental Health program at the hospital. They'll hook you up with a psychiatrist who will analyze your situation." He warned me that not everyone could take Citalopram in the daytime, and I may have to take it at night, which proved to be the case.

[Citalopram is an antidepressant used to treat depression and anxiety disorders and I would later switch to Escitalopram; a similar medication with fewer side effects.]

That first dose left me stoned. I'd spent the entire day on my couch, higher than a kite, and I tried to focus on something, anything. The trees swaying in the breeze outside my living room window had me mesmerized—the leaves twirling, lulling me to sleep, curled up with a pillow and throw. The next day, I switched it up and took it with my evening pills. I slept like the dead. After a few weeks, it kicked in—my mental state had improved, but I felt dopier than ever. My speech slowed and became stilted. The right words were tough to find. 'Um' appeared in every sentence.

By then I'd tired of lazing around and sitting inside, looking out at beautiful sunny fall days. I forced myself to go out walking short distances, using cabs and buses when fatigued and couldn't walk anymore. October moved into November, and the weather turned. No walking down steep hills to the beach like I had back in April. The air was crisp, and the rain clouds blew in and stayed. Their drops showered the earth, drenching everything in their path.

A year after my stay at the Sullivan District Hilton, as I referred to it, my mind remained befuddled. I still heard the ringing of silent phones, music and voices that belonged to no one, and rooms and nature that moved past me as though riding atop a conveyor belt. Flickering lights like glittering tear drops tinkled down the outer edges of my peripheral vision. First one eye and then the other. They took turns in their quest to drive me to madness. Weird sensations of a hand that caressed the back of my neck or of glasses resting on top of my head which had lain on the table in front of me. Even my other senses had conspired against me. I could not write legibly, my fingers stiff, as if petrified. My lack of eye hand coordination caused a clumsiness far greater than before. I'd reach out to grasp a glass from the cupboard, a door handle, or a bag only to knock over, drop or miss them entirely. My exceptional balance disappeared, and left me grabbing handrails, leaning against walls and posts just to maintain my equilibrium. Loud noises and fast movements, combined with my balance issues, had made walking along busy roadways a challenge. Noise cancelling headphones had eased part of the problem, and the music masked the roar of engines and honking horns. Nothing could stop the blur that'd whizzed past me—a smear of colours that blended form and structure into a jumbled mess.

*\*\*November 2016 Bus Incident No. 1\*\**

I went shopping at Walmart to cheer myself up. I purchased matching towels, face cloths, and a new shower curtain for the main bathroom. My family cautioned me not to spend too much money updating my home. 'You don't know how long you'll be off work. You can't burn through your savings.' And so on. So I appeased myself by buying minor items to change the look and feel, creating an illusion that more had taken place. As would happen often, I'd gotten carried away and bought too much to carry the thirty minutes to home and had opted to take the bus.

I clamoured aboard and sat behind the driver, my parcels beside me. His seat blocked the view of the road ahead, limiting the scenery that whizzed by. Whether because of the cocktail of meds or the temporal resection or both, I couldn't stare out the window of a moving vehicle. The speed at which the houses, trees, lampposts, and cars would pass by—distorted. My mind visualized the movement fifty times faster than it was.

As we jostled along, turning corners and waiting at stoplights, I stared at the driver's seat. My iPod played my 80s favourites, floating from one to another, my foot tapping to the beat. It was only another two blocks to my stop and another two to walk home.

I exited, took a few steps, and placed my bags on the bench as I surveyed my surroundings. I glanced at the direction we had come from and turned and stared at the rear of the bus as it rumbled away. The trees and bushes weren't familiar. The shapes and where they stood seemed different. Even the houses looked new to me. I didn't know where I was or which way to go. My heart raced. All I could hear was a thumping in my ears as though a beating drum was inside me. It was not until I spied the partially constructed house on the corner that I knew where I was and that I would be okay.—'Ah. *That is where I must go.*' I crossed the street and trekked down the road, the area becoming familiar as I went. The sight of my front steps released the tension that had coiled around my shoulders. I made it home.

As I kicked off my shoes and dumped my bag on the floor, I felt deflated. What had been a fun outing—destroyed. Those few moments that transported me to the darkness and confusion had spoiled my enjoyment from shopping. Disgusted, angry, and sad, I threw my purchases down the stairs to the basement. I had been eager to wash and hang the new towels and shower curtain, but the desire had gone. I couldn't be bothered. Not knowing where I was had frightened me. It had felt surreal–like a dream or a scary movie and had left me feeling vulnerable. I curled up on the couch and cried myself to sleep.

It was then I believed the depression and anxiety had taken hold of my fragile spirit. From then onwards, I'd viewed the world from the safety of my nest. I created walls and had kept the light out. I'd become numb, unwilling to feel positive about anything. Angry and resentful. Pangs of jealousy and rage welled up against those who didn't have a demon inside controlling their lives. Those feelings took hold over the days, creating a false reality. Deep below the surface I'd known I needed help, the kind that those close to me couldn't provide.

And so I began a search for some support. There had to be some groups out there to help others like me. I was fighting a daily battle alone, frightened, and with no one to talk to that could relate to my experiences. I needed something, anything. Someone who didn't know me but knew all about epilepsy.

It took some time before I found two organisations that I thought could help. Neither one was close to home. One group devoted to education and awareness wasn't accessible by bus, but I emailed, asking if there were any groups closer to me I could join. They never responded. My email went unanswered. What use was an organisation offering education and awareness if they ignored you? I then found a listing for the BC Epilepsy Society in Vancouver and asked them if they knew of any groups close to me. Yes, they did. They had a support group in Vancouver that met once a month in the evening. It would take two buses and the SkyTrain plus ten minutes of walking to reach their offices. I wouldn't travel outside my community by myself and had had no one available to accompany me. My situation had seemed hopeless until they told me about their online group. They referred me to the group coordinator, and in December, I took part in my first session.

Through a conferencing computer program called Zoom, I could see and speak to others as if in the same room. I stared at the computer screen, talked and listened to others going through the same things I was. I'd felt like a child attending his first birthday party. My body buzzed with excitement. I laughed and smiled. To have connected with a group of men and women that could relate to the same issues I'd been having encouraged me. I'd found a safe place where I could speak without judgement. Discussions on what medications we'd all tried, which worked and those which didn't. The methods used to reduce stress were helpful.

With each session, I felt my fears and anxieties weaken and the depressive state I'd been in turn around and I no longer felt lonely. I'd gotten more out of those sessions than from the shrink I'd seen the year before. What puzzled me was how none of my doctors had spoken of the Epilepsy Society. That no one talked about this valuable resource available to those struggling to manage this incurable disease. It was as if the Epilepsy Society didn't exist. My doctors hadn't even offered any other forms of therapy or support networks I could access to help cope with the challenges I faced. They had left it up to me to seek these out, to ask Google. The Medical System had let me down yet again.

*On December 16, 2016,* I went to see Dr. Edwards for my next follow-up appointment.

"Merry Christmas, Ms. McClure, how have you been feeling? Any more incidents on buses?"

"Merry Christmas to you too, Dr. Edwards. Did you have a wonderful holiday?"

"Yes, thank you. I see from your tracking calendar those pains and headaches seem to have increased along with your waves. Can you tell me more about your bus experience and the pains you're having?"

"Yeah, um, these pains are like, um, like a headache, but not quite. It's constant, and then I get these sharp jabs like a knife going into my head." I patted the right side up at the incision site and down at the temple.

"How long do those last? The jabs? How strong are they on a scale of 1 to 10, ten being the worst?"

"They don't last long, and are quite, um, strong. It feels like..8 or 9?"

"Okay." He sat back in his chair, his brow furrowed. He tapped his pen on the desk and glanced at his computer screen, then at me, and back again. Setting the pen aside, he leaned forward, placed his arms on the desk, clasped his hands and looked up at me. "What I'm going to suggest we do, if it's alright with you, is to put you on Gabapentin. We prescribe it for pain, but it also has some anti-seizure properties. Minor, mind you, but with your other meds, it would add another layer to help control things." Not waiting for my answer, he scribbled on his prescription pad, ripped a page off and handed it to me. "Now, tell me about this blanking out on the bus." He sat back and placed his elbows on the armrests and waited.

"Yeah, um, I was coming home from shopping... and I felt confused after. Um, it was like I was there, but really wasn't, you know? Like I knew I was on a bus, and there were people around me, but I was, um, like not aware they were there? Does that make sense?" As I spoke, he sat up, made some notes, nodded and smiled.

"Let's get you going on the Gabapentin and see what that does for the pains. I want to order an MRI." He turned to me as he spoke. *Interesting. I knew he would want to do one. Could feel it in my gut.* I had to ask him to repeat the last part. Lost in my thoughts, I had missed what he said.

"I want to be sure that nothing has changed to the skullcap at the incision site—that it hasn't shifted. I'm also going to have you do an overnight Oximeter test. I want to rule out sleep apnea as a potential cause for your tiredness. Once that's done, I'll have you come back for a follow-up."

**December 2016 Bus Incident No. 2**

Dr. Patrick, my GP, had been an enormous support for Devon and me during this time. So much so, we purchased a gift to show our appreciation.

It was only a half-hour bus trip. That day was crisp and sunny, the air filled with the aroma of smoke from fireplaces and soggy leaves rotting in composts. The icy blue green water of Mud Bay with the Northshore Mountains in the background beckoned us. A walk along the promenade would do us both good. We settled into our seats on the bus and headed off. Dev was a row behind and across the aisle. I relaxed against the headrest. Happy thoughts of giving to others and a walk along one of my favourite beaches calmed my mind. I don't know at what point my conscious slipped into a slumber. I have vague recollections of right turns and a left that wander into my memories, drifting among a wispy fog. It was normal for the bus to announce each upcoming stop, allowing passengers the time to ring the bell. I can recall hearing Anderson Street, but nothing afterwards.

Twenty blocks later, as new passengers boarded, my eyes opened. I'd looked around me, searching for something familiar. I hadn't known where I was at first, had been confused. It'd taken a few moments before I'd realized where I was. "OH. We're here in Ocean Park," I muttered to myself. I had been oblivious as we'd passed houses, stores, pedestrians, and cars. Dev seated behind me had witnessed nothing out of the ordinary.

I continued glancing around, bringing myself back into the present, when a sickly sweet stench filled my nostrils. *Pot so strong I wanted to retch.* A man seated across the aisle held a backpack between his legs. He wore a wool coat that looked as though it had had a battle with shears and lost. It was too small for him. The seams pulled and stretched and the buttons strained to hold it closed. His toque, barely containing the greasy tangled curls, sat askew, threatening to fall off. The stench that assaulted my poor nose rose from his bundle. It wafted across the aisle like steam from a kettle, floating upwards and filling the surrounding air. It'd smelt like skunk spray, powerful and disgusting, so strong even Devon detected it from two seats away. Our stop couldn't have arrived soon enough.

I'd made light of my 'blank out' by blaming the fumes that had drifted across to me and impairing my senses. But as with my adventure the previous month, we couldn't determine if I'd had a simple partial seizure or an instance of just not paying attention. Either way, both incidents had required further investigation.

Months passed by and I experienced no further zoning out episodes, but found the effects from sitting sideways on buses and looking out the windows amplified the distortion. Daylight peeping in between the trees and houses emitted a strobe-like effect. Their erratic flashing scrambled my brain, sending it into overload. I couldn't process the rapid fluctuations of light and scenery. The rapid fire movements too fast. Their effects were like shaking a snow globe, disturbing the white flecks into a swirling mass twirling around an image encased in glass.

*We'd all been so sure of a positive outcome. That the surgery would be a success and I'd be on my way towards a seizure-free life - my future had been bright. But when those signs had shown the opposite, it'd stunned everyone, had baffled my doctors, and knocked me down.*

*Best laid plans. What a crock of shit.*

# PART THREE

## *** 2017—2018—Commuting to Alberta***

## Chapter Eleven

***February 10, 2017—Check-Up—Dr. Edwards' Office, Surrey, BC***

I'd arrived early and stood at reception waiting to check in. The young lady behind the desk had just hung up the phone. She turned in her chair towards me and smiled.

"Hi Angela, I got the date for my MRI today." I'd held up the notice I received in the mail. "Are you ready for this?"Angela leaned back in her chair, crossed her arms, and waited, her eyes intent on the piece of paper I held. "Ok, here it is. August 2019. Two and a half years from now. Can you believe it?" I moved it closer so she could read the date highlighted in yellow.

"Oh, Linda. I'm sorry. That's outrageous. You're the first patient we've had whose appointment goes beyond 2018. I don't know what to say?"

Neither did I.

My follow-up with Dr. Edwards was a quick one. We reviewed the results of the CT Scan from December 22, 2016, and the Oximeter test. All had come back normal.

"Oh, I had another blank out before Christmas. Dev was with me but didn't see it." I described the bus trip and how I didn't recall the route from uptown to Ocean Park.

"So, we don't know for sure, but these could only be a case of being unaware of what's going on around you. For example, when you're driving along and the next thing you know, you've arrived at your destination. That's normal for anyone and happens from time to time. In your situation, it would be more commonplace for several reasons. Your epilepsy for one, and the side effects of the drugs and after-effects of the surgery." He ticked off his fingers with each one as he spoke. "I'm not saying that's happening. Or that they're seizure-related, but we don't want to jump the gun and come to any conclusions yet."

***Journal Entry, February 11, 2017***

*My Oximeter test came back normal. Dr. Edwards was testing for sleep apnea. I don't have it. Thank God. The pains have continued despite the Gabapentin. I'm at the max dose— 3x day. and I take Extra Strength Tylenol or Advil if it's terrible. I had another weird thing occur late January, to which I refer to as my puppet arm. Dr. Edwards does not believe it's seizure related. I saw him yesterday with Dev. First time Dev has met him. After all, Dev lives with me and whether he realizes it, he may be the only witness to any odd behaviour I may have. I know it's hard on him. He has to deal with this at his age when he has his own shit going on. I feel useless, like I've failed him. I'm all he's got. He's had no male influence in his life. Mom was involved with Margaret and her girls, and Jim was too far away. Now, when Devon's finally dealing with all those inner feelings and emotions he's buried for so long, I'm helpless and a burden to him. I don't remember a lot of stuff. I'm mixing up or forgetting words and using the wrong ones. I'm finding it hard to make simple decisions and can't handle stressful situations. I try to rely on my organizational skills, but it's hard when you forget what you're doing or can't focus for too long. Everything takes way longer than it used to. Takes more effort. Dr. Edwards is sending me for an MRI and EEG—a check-up, you could say—checking things out under the hood to see if all the plugs and wires connected are firing right. Too late. Hahaha. They burnt out and fried up long before now.*

*\*\*February 15, 2017—Face-to-face follow up with Dr. Young–*

*Calgary\*\**

As part of Dr. Young's post surgical follow up, he requested I fly in—easier to gauge my progress in person than over the phone. It was the first time I'd seen him outside of the seizure unit.

"Hi, Dr. Young, this is my son, Devon." We went through a brief introduction and how are you while we took our seats. We gathered our papers and pens and settled down to business.

"Ms. McClure. I see from Dr. Edwards's notes that you've been experiencing events that may or may not be seizure-related. I nodded. How many of these waves do you have per day or week?"

"It varies." I rummaged through my bag and pulled out a worn manila file folder. "I prepared these notes to give you an idea of what's going on, and I've included copies of the calendars I do for Dr. Edwards. I wasn't sure if he'd passed them onto you." After scanning them and updating my meds, he sat back. He peered at me over the rim of his glasses, a thoughtful expression upon his face.

"I want to bring you back into the seizure unit, if I may? I want to determine if these events are seizures or not. The only way to be certain is to bring you back in for monitoring. Are you up for that?" I nodded and grinned.

"I suspected that would be the next step. Yes. If coming back is going to figure this all out, then yes, I'm all for it. But let me warn you, Dr. Young. I'm not 'normal' with medical stuff." I held up both hands, making air quotes to emphasize my lack of normalcy. "Like when I had my hysterectomy, all the tests had shown nothing. What they found were fibroids, cysts on my ovaries, endometriosis and adenomyosis." I stopped to catch my breath. "I had everything and anything that could've been going and then some. As my old boss used to say, I don't do easy."

Shaking his head, he stared at me, across the desk, and back at me without uttering a word.

"Ok, we will be in touch with you once there's an opening in the unit." Dr. Young uncrossed his legs and pushed his chair back, signalling an end to my visit. "Try some relaxation techniques to reduce your stress and anxiety. We'll see you back here in a few months. Take care of yourself, Ms. McClure." He scooped up his papers and exited the room. I'd either embarrassed him by speaking of my woman's plumbing, or he had a busy day ahead, which prompted his quick departure.

### **Me Vs Ministry of Health**

I couldn't fill my Clobazam prescription. There was a supply shortage. I emailed the Health Ministry and informed them of my plight.

*Dear Sir,*

*I am writing to you based on an article found in The Toronto Star titled: "Canada-wide shortage of epilepsy drug reaches 'crisis' point".*

*I informed him I was one of the 20,000-40,000 who relied on this drug to manage my epilepsy. That my pharmacist was*

178

*out of supply and couldn't help me. I told him my seizures weren't being controlled with the four drugs I take and reducing it to three would be disastrous. I described my seizures, and the many trips to the emergency room, and pointed out the drain on the medical system because my seizures were out of control. I went on about the lack of resources in BC and the inadequately equipped seizure unit. How I've had to go to Alberta to seek help and the cost to me to do so. The lack of awareness and research and education about epilepsy. And on.*

*\*\*Their Response\*\**

*Dear Ms. McClure:*

*We're sorry to read about the health challenges with your seizures. They thanked me for my comments about access to neurologists specialising in seizure disorders.*

*(The usual government rhetoric about the many contributing factors, shortages of materials, process problems, suppliers, quality control, and so on followed this.)*

*We're collaborating with other provinces, the industry, practitioners, and we track shortages as they occur. Clobazam is being monitored closely. Contact your doctor about changing your other prescriptions.*

After receiving my MRI appointment for August 2019, I sent another email.

*Today I am writing to you about the ridiculous wait times for necessary tests such as MRIs. It was my understanding you addressed this issue and were increasing hours of operation.* I stated that either it hadn't happened yet, or the process wasn't working, and informed him of my MRI appointment scheduled two-and-a-half years from then. I explained the reason for it. The surgery, pains, headaches, and the concern of postoperative complications. That I had to go to Calgary because of our broken system. That the ministry let me down, and I'd lost faith in them.

The purpose of the MRI was to determine if the pains and headaches since my surgery were because the Krazy-Glue hadn't kept the skull plate in place, or was my discomfort from healing nerve endings? The backlog of patients waiting for MRIs and CT scans and lengthy wait times were news du jour. There wasn't a TV or radio station or newspaper that didn't cover the story. Social media was ablaze with comments and accusations. Besides wait-times, many patients faced drug shortages, and I fell under both categories. Thus, I began my 'medical email-rant' as I referred to it:

On February 24, 2017, I emailed the Health Minister and copied my representatives of Parliament and Legislative Assembly.

*Dear Sir,*

*Today I am writing to you about the ridiculous wait times that continue for British Columbians for necessary tests such as MRI's.*

*It was my understanding that this issue was and had been addressed by increasing the hours of running these tests. Either this has not been implemented yet, as the government and media had reported it, or the process isn't working.*

I went on to inform him of my MRI appointment scheduled 2 ½ years from then. I explained the reason for it. The surgery, pains, headaches, and the concern of post-operative complications. That I had to go to Calgary because the system here was broken. That the ministry let me down and I'd lost faith in them.

This time, to be sure my voice carried loud and clear, I sent copies to the medical authority and the opposition's health critic.

My first reply was from the health critic. She was quite interested in my story. The Opposition had the health minister running for cover as they attacked on all fronts, demanding change. Emails were exchanged, a copy of my appointment notice scanned and forwarded, showing proof of my lengthy wait.

The medical authority replied next with their tales of woe. After increasing the MRI capacity, they still experienced significant wait times for non-urgent requests. Their fix was to send me to other locations with shorter wait times. Reasonable, yes, except for one who doesn't drive. Two of the three locations weren't accessible by bus and were more than an hour away. The third required three buses or more. Not an easy feat for one doped up on four drugs, single, with no one available to take me. It was obvious they didn't understand the scope of how disabling epilepsy was.

With my permission, the health critic brought up my story during the House of Commons Question Period on March 7, 2017.

Cross-legged on the floor, ears and eyes open, watching the proceedings. Back and forth, they went, health critic to health minister, my name echoing in the hall each time they spoke. My story was on radio and social media. The official transcripts, a permanent record on file found on the internet.

https://www.leg.bc.ca/content/Hansard/40th6th/20170307 am-Hansard-v43n1.htm

Even now, when I Google my name, my story can be found on websites outside of Canada; for advertising from private imaging companies and services. News of how poorly our health system was operating to the detriment of all patients had spread.

The Health Ministry's response came almost a month after the House was in session.

They were sorry for my health issues. Timely access to imaging is important and they were working to address the long wait times. A plan was in place with new funding to provide 65,000 more scans by 2019. It was all just a repeat of what the health minister stated throughout the question period. We've added this. We're doing that. But, sorry we can't help you in your time of need.

**March 18, 2017, Journal Entry**

*Not a pleasant week. I had a seizure on Monday, March 13. Heh. Almost 2 years to the day since the one that started all this. Go figure. It was pretty fucking scary, though. I don't like these seizures where I know what's going on. The other ones were scary cause I hadn't known what I'd been doing and I could've gotten hurt. But, knowing what's going on and being helpless and alone and not being able to call for help or get to medication... I think that's WAY WORSE.*

My frame of mind was the polar opposite of how it had been two years ago. That first seizure in 2015 left me afraid to be alone and I wouldn't go out by myself. This time, I'd felt safer outside. Being among others was better than staying in where no one could see or hear me. Thoughts of a repeat performance made me tremble, break out in a cold sweat: tension builds and chest tightens as fear takes hold. As a precaution, I gave keys to my neighbours and exchanged phone numbers should I need help. Life moved along. I refused to let this seizure ruin all my hard work—couldn't let it set me back. I was determined to get through the remainder of March without further incident. I made adjustments here and there, tweaking the processes to fit my ever-changing, developing illness. And then the ghostly images and tinkling lights began.

I stared at my ceiling fan, slow to open my eyes from a dream-filled night. I shifted my eyes to the night table in search of my phone. All I saw was the fan cast in a ghostly shadow. Other objects around the room produced the same eerie images. Pictures hanging on the wall, the curtain rod, closet, dresser, all the same. Déjà vu transported me back to 2015, and the overexposed body image was in the doorway of my hospital room. The ghostly images escalated to doorframes, chairs, and my cat, occurring first thing in the morning, throughout the day and into the evening. In my notes, I called them Ghost Images—no other explanation could describe them. A month later, the 'light thingy' started. Dotted lights that would trickle around my line of vision. Starting near the top of my eye, cascading over to the side and down. Miniature diamonds shimmering in the light and trickling down like water droplets.

*** Journal entry—April 1, 2017***

*Life has resumed its "hurry up and wait for the phone to ring" lifestyle that I've become accustomed to for the last couple of years.*

*' What if I couldn't have reached my phone?' runs through my mind every-once-in-a-while.*

*So, my mixing up word thing is still happening. Called up to Dev the other day—"You up? Thought I heard footprints?" Hmm... how do you hear prints?? Oh, damn it! I mean footsteps!*

*Oh, and apparently, my mind can turn a garbage bag into Coco. It's done that a couple of times. AND! I can turn Dev's bag into a Calico cat who sits on the dining room table cleaning its paws!! Pretty cool, eh? The word thing and Coco being a garbage bag was happening before this last seizure. But the Calico cat thing was after. All the "visions" seemed so vivid, real.*

*There are some wires crossed or shorting out up in my head. Something just isn't right. The surgery may have gone well, but maybe the healing process isn't? I don't know. I hope Dr. Young can get a better idea of what's going on in this freaky head of mine. I did warn him. I told him I wasn't normal, especially when it comes to this kind of stuff!*

***SMU—Take Two—'Camp Seizure Unit'***

By this time, I was a pro. It was my third trip to Foothills Medical Centre in Calgary and, being familiar with the routine and staff, smiling and joking, I'd sauntered past the nurses' station, around the corner and through the blue-painted door into the SMU. SMU was how the staff referenced the seizure monitoring unit, and I'd adopted their lingo—a normal progression considering I was fast becoming a regular.

"Wow, I get a window seat this time? *Cool.*" A larger room. One wall of windows with a view of the helicopter landing pad and surrounding hillside. No mountain views. Only rolling hills (oversized molehills to a BC girl), dotted with houses, trees, and roadways. A ledge ran the length of the windows with room enough for my suitcase, books, and snacks. I took out what I needed, changed into my Foothills attire, and waited. It was Olivia this time who walked me down the corridor to attach my electrodes. We chatted about the weather, living in BC, and my health. Back in my room, high off the fumes of the glue, we began hooking me up. Cables and wires plugged into the Walkman-sized gizmo placed into the stylish pouch. The jeopardy button tucked into place.

"Test:" a press of the button and the bell sprang to life. All good. Now we sit and wait. Wait for the electrical storms to short-circuit my neurons—creating sparks of lightning unique to me.

**Journal Entry June 2017**

*I arrived on the 22nd, and it took three days to produce a seizure similar to the March 13th event minus the shaking. I felt wavey, anxious, tired and endured head pains. The room spun. Arms and legs tingled, and I felt spacey, floating almost. The trickling lights returned, as did the waves, lots of waves. My poor head felt banged up—battered night and day. Sharp pains, eyes sore. Tired.*

**Journal Entry June 26, 2017**

*My drugs are now down to almost nothing. Only half of my Lamotrigine dose and my Dilantin is all that remains. Over the last couple of days, I've had more waves than I care to count. I think I've had more waves in the last few days than I've had in some months. They wear my body out. My legs, especially. With each of the seizures, my legs felt cemented to the bed. No jerking or shaking, just 2 long useless limbs — dead and not listening to the commander in charge… my beat-up brain. My arms were shaky and feeble, but not as noodle-like as my legs. I feel like I've run for days and dropped to my hands and knees for the last mile. Fortunately, my body was in the game and performed nicely for the SPECT Scan. Wave followed by a seizure. Now I glow in the dark from the radioactive dye injected into me to illuminate the area the seizures originated from. (I wondered if I still need a night light at home?). The plan is to still kick me out and send me flying home on Thursday. My meds are being increased again as of tonight, and I get a day of rest as no tests scheduled for tomorrow. The idea is to redo the SPECT with no seizure activity to compare with the one I had today. Hence, the increase to my meds tonight and tomorrow. Wednesday is SPECT day, and Thursday is MRI. Before I head to home sweet home, there will be a discussion about surgery should that be our course of action. Surgery, sigh, again. I must reset the clock on 1. nerve healing 2. pain 3. my hair 4. exercise 5. coming off any of my meds. Sigh. If this is the next step and brings me closer to having a more normal life, then I guess it's what I need to do. I seem/feel strangely calm about it. Interesting. Probably because I've been through it already and know what to expect. Or maybe the fact that it's a more straightforward surgery, for them, cause there's already a pathway there — so no big deal, right? It's just like walking through deep snow. The first time is hard as you put your foot into the virgin snow. As it gets trampled, the easier it is to move and see where to go.*

**Journal Entry June 28, 2017**

*I was back to full dose on meds. WAVES milder now-back to normal. Headaches persisted. SPECT Scan #2 now completed.*

Dr. O'Connor, one neurologist on the team, explained their findings.

I can picture him standing beside my bed, drawing pictures on the whiteboard as he described the various areas of concern in my brain. Just as with all the other doctors I'd come in contact with, he looked younger than he was. Of average build, short dark hair, his gaze gentle and kind, his voice soft, almost soothing, his smile genuine. The team had determined I'd return for intracranial monitoring. They would insert tiny wires into my brain to get closer to the source of my troubles. All my test results had concluded a light still burned at the end of the tunnel where they'd removed part of the temporal lobe ten months earlier. Its lumens shone and pulsed, proving that more digging was necessary. Preliminary tests had also revealed a second war that'd raged in what's called the Insula. What they couldn't determine was if the Insula acted up on its own, or was the remaining lesion sending off signals for the second wave of attack? Or was it vice versa? Was one of them the instigator and the other following behind? By sticking the electrodes into the brain tissue, we'd get a front-row seat to capture those events.

*__Journal Entry June 30, 2017__*

*Discharged yesterday. Tired, and dopier being back on a full dose of meds, I flew home.*

*August 29, 2017*

I was in the kitchen making my lunch when a massive wave hit. After a couple of minutes, a seizure started. My arms tingled; the nerves vibrated. I felt dopey and lightheaded. It moved down my legs–the sensation within them drained away like a plugged up sink that trickled down the blocked pipes. My hands grabbed underneath the counter. My feet couldn't move. They felt as if they'd turned to stone. When my arm shook and my hold on the counter had loosened, I called out to Devon for help. He laid me down, gave me an Ativan, and started a timer. If the seizure hadn't stopped after five minutes, he'd call for an ambulance. We'd learned by then that seizing for over five minutes reduced the amount of oxygen to the brain. Uncontrolled seizures lasting longer than five minutes could cause serious brain damage, even death.

The paramedics arrived and administered more Ativan, bundled me up onto the stretcher, and whisked me off to the hospital. I remember rubbing my forehead, temples, sides. They'd throbbed with pain far worse than any normal headache.

[Postictal headaches are all-encompassing. A steady or throbbing pain ranging from mild to severe that can last between about 6 and 24 hours, or more.]

192

The nurse had said the paramedics estimated the seizure had lasted 25-30 minutes based on when Devon placed the 911 call. Once I'd been able to walk and use the bathroom, the doctor released me. It was 8pm by the time we'd arrived home and almost 9pm before I crawled into bed. By lunch time the next day, the veil lifted, and functionality returned. Except the fingers. Stiff from the blip, not fully reset, they could not even hold a pen. Movement across the page was shaky, the words almost illegible. My notes were choppy, almost senseless. As my body rebooted, an immense tiredness set in. Muscles and tendons, weary from tension, had felt battered. Bruised by the sensations that had attacked them.

Anxiety and depression, a common by-product of epilepsy, and the fear of reoccurring seizures and side effects had altered my state of mind. Dr. Patrick submitted a referral to the mental health program back in the spring, but it'd taken until summer to get into a support group. Navigating through the mental health system is a long process: a waiting period to see a psychiatrist, a second referral, and then another waitlist. My road to freedom from anxiety began in March, but it'd taken until August to get into Cognitive Behaviour Therapy. The group sessions had proved ineffective for me. They were not designed for someone with my comprehension and cognitive dysfunctions. Sitting in a circle among others with varying degrees of problems and symptoms, I was an outsider. Most had a relationship or work concerns, some both. I was the square peg trying to fit into a round hole. Sent away each week with homework to complete, taking turns reading the weekly lessons out loud, increased my stress and anxiety instead of easing them. What I needed, what my doctors wanted, was individual therapy. The system couldn't provide that. I persevered through three of the four weeks, then stopped. I'd had a seizure the day before the last session and couldn't attend.

*\*\*Me vs the Minister of Mental Health and Addictions\*\**

In my second round of ranting, I directed in an email to the Minister of Mental Health and Addictions with a copy to the BC Health Minister. I described my need for therapy and the progression from referral to therapy and the six months I'd gone without the help I was desperate to find. I explained that I'd had comprehension and cognitive deficiencies and needed the same individual support like stroke patients. I mentioned that I had many of the same challenges since my surgery, but had to seek help privately at the cost of $100 or more per session. I informed the Minister how the BC Epilepsy Society, my only free resource, had its government funding cut. How access to individuals who know what epilepsy is, and what one goes through, had now shrunk, limiting the availability of the few medical professionals with training and knowledge to provide that support. I briefly outlined my struggle to control my seizures and maintain a healthy mental state and dealing with the stigma surrounding epilepsy that still exists increases the anxieties and depression—fostering a state of loneliness and isolation. Pointed out that I'm just one of the thousands of individuals in BC that go without the necessary resources, support, and access to qualified doctors.

I couldn't deny that they weren't trying to improve the system, but, for me, it hadn't been soon enough. *Talking* about hiring more doctors and nurse practitioners is not the same as *doing*. They couldn't force students into medical training, nor could they place them in remote areas to provide better access to medical care. This 'team-based approach' they'd tossed around like confetti was a grand concept, in theory. But to implement it would take time.

The Ministry's response came two months later:

The usual, we are sorry for your situation.

We know there is a problem and have a mandate to improve things

We're going to do this and do that

We have a 5-year plan

Your input is valuable

Their response to my costs to commute between provinces for care was to quote policy I already knew. The government's remedy to my search for a neuropsychologist was to send a website link to low-cost therapy options through counsellors and therapists. They hadn't understood my need for specialized care and the limited resources they offered to treat epilepsy.

I'm fortunate to have a family that helped me get the care I need. Family members to escort me back and forth, contribute to my expenses, and provide me with a place to stay when needed. Others not so lucky continue to suffer while years pass by. My little voice was whistling past their ears, carried away

196

by the wind. I tried reaching out to the media after my moment in the spotlight. But that too fell on deaf ears. I was no longer newsworthy, and I suspect they felt epilepsy didn't affect many people, so who cared?

*[I've always said you can only beat your head against a wall for so long before giving up.  And I let this one go and moved on.]*

# Chapter Twelve

## **Drilling and Surgery SMU Take Three—

## 'Foothills Chateau'**

*November 2017 Intracranial Monitoring—My Medusa Look*

Home again and life is in limbo, waiting for the call to book my craniotomy in the fall. My sister Margaret would travel with me for the surgery scheduled for November 3rd. However, thanks to Hurricane Irma, a replacement part for the machine necessary for the operation was slow to come out of Florida and the operation got pushed back to November 7th. Another call from Foothills altered our dates once more. I hadn't completed the memory retest a year after my August surgery, and they wouldn't proceed without having it done. They booked me for November 1st and 2nd. Which meant we had to leave on October 31st, two days earlier than planned. Margaret wasn't impressed with the shifting dates. She'd had a trip to Palm Springs later that month, and if my stay required more than a couple of weeks, she'd have to cancel and pay a fee. I'd told her to just dump and run. That she didn't need to stay. After all, I'd been at the SMU alone before and had managed just fine. But she came, and it all worked out.

With both the preoperative exam and memory test completed, we'd had the weekend to ourselves. November 3rd was our brother Jim's 55th birthday, and we'd spent it at his home in Red Deer. It had been the first time in over 20 years that the three of us had been under one roof together. We'd had a lovely weekend full of laughter and quality time with family, playing cards and eating home-cooked food.

*\*\*November 6, 2017–Craniotomy Step One: The Mask\*\**

They placed a 'cage' on my head—a back catcher's mask, but sturdier with thick metal bars. Two pieces bolted to my head after freezing injected to forehead, temples, and at the back where screws fastened the cage in place. Sitting, hands in my lap, cracking jokes with my sister and a surgical resident from Dr. Taylor's team, my Frankenstein transformation progressed. Over to the MRI machine, I sat on the table for step two. They placed a shield over my head. Thinking that was it, I'd swung my legs up and onto the table, prepared to get settled before sliding into the tube. This process wasn't new to me. I'd done it countless times before, minus the hardware.

"Ok, Linda, sit still. We're going to place this on top. It's heavy, so we must support your head as you lie down."

A second technologist had entered the room carrying a white helmet similar to what an astronaut might have worn. I twisted my body to get a better look at this additional piece of hardware. I'd felt like a Storm Trooper. With the resident helping in front and the technologist in back, they laid me down, supporting my head as they went. Heavy was an understatement. If they had let go, my neck would snap in half as easy as a stick of spaghetti.

"Now, let us shift you into position; don't move by yourself."

Inch by inch, we moved up the table, and they placed my head into the cradle. Confident that I was in the correct position and comfortable, they set the shield in place. I lay there, breathing in and out for what seemed like hours. The banging inside the tube vibrated throughout my body, a steady rhythmic beat that was soothing to me.

"That was great, Linda; we're all done. Don't move. Wait for us to help you up."

They lead me back to my sister and my 'chariot.' I settled in place. After a brief wait, the porter arrived to wheel me up to the OR. The cage would remain until the surgery was over. It was a guide to assist the surgeon with placing the electrodes. Transferred to the OR table, and with local freezing in place, I heard the whir of a drill. I would be awake during the procedure.

"Here we go, Linda. Let me know if you feel anything, and we'll put more freezing in, Ok?" Dr. Taylor said as he'd readied himself to proceed.

"Yup, okey-dokey."

I felt the pressure of the bit against my skull. The whine of the drill with further pressure told me it had started. In and out it went along the side, a bit in back and a few on top for good measure. I couldn't keep from visualizing the skin tearing apart, the grinding of bone, as the blood-splattered drill pushed through. The whole experience was surreal, felt like a scene from a horror flick. I was in and out in what seemed like a short time and was returned to my cell just as the lunch tray arrived.

My head now bandaged up, we returned to the unit. Olivia wasted no time attaching the wires and cables. She wrapped my head, turban style, in a gauze-like tension bandage but much lighter. I looked like a bleached-out Hershey Kiss.

My head felt as if someone tapped a nail setter into my head, trying to smooth out the surface of my skull. It didn't take long before flares erupted. Mobility was more of a challenge than the first time. Where before I only had a 'leash' to deal with, this time, I had a 'buddy.' With wires poked into my brain, cables ran to a box on wheels, which attached to a cord that ran to the computer mounted high on the wall. My 'buddy' came with me each time I visited the toilet, or went anywhere. Wheels attached to legs like a steno chair caught on the table tray, the bed, doors and tangled up the cords. Negotiating around these obstacles was like pushing a shopping cart one-handed with a wobbly wheel. It took a few days, but I got the hang of my 'shopping cart.' I used the little wire basket attached below the box to hold my bathroom items that reduced the number of trips there and back. It held toothpaste and brush, face cloth and towel, soap, deodorant, face cream, and snacks. Parked beside my bed, it made an impromptu night table that allowed me access to necessities without tangling up cords and wires while I manoeuvred around my cramped space.

One day I'd caught Dr. Young and Dr. Joseph standing across the unit, hands covering their grinning faces, stifling the sounds of laughter at the picture I presented. I was leaving the bathroom with my 'shopping cart' in tow, its basket filled with toiletries and other sundries. I glanced at the pair and had known what they'd been thinking,

"Yeah, I know. I look like a bag lady, don't I?" I'd called out.

They couldn't contain themselves any longer; their laughter erupted, leaving me shaking my head as I wheeled into my cave. Despite the struggles my body had gone through, I'd kept my sense of humour.

All four beds held patients from outside of Alberta: my neighbour from Manitoba, a girl from the Maritimes, and a fellow next to her hailed from BC. Conversations conducted from our doorways had helped the days flow. Being the curious beast I was, it was interesting to hear about other forms of epilepsy different to mine. How, unlike me, one lady only had seizures in her sleep. A scary concept to me compared to mine. That no one would know you were seizing unless it alerted your spouse or other family member to your movements. It made my seizures almost trivial and less risky.

Two days after they had implanted the wires, I'd had a seizure. It'd started just after dinner. I'd had problems pushing food around in my mouth–shifting it towards the back of my mouth to the throat. When I'd taken a sip of water to clear the mass, it dribbled down and onto my bib. The left side had drooped and the water, mixed with saliva, seeped out and down my chin. My speech became slurred and words wouldn't come out. It'd carried on for over five minutes. When I hadn't been able to move my legs and the arms had become heavy and inert, the nurse administered Ativan. As it progressed, I'd lost awareness but could perform simple tasks–or so I'd been told. When the doctors made their rounds the next morning, they informed me that the seizure had lasted for three hours. I'd gone into status epilepticus.

*[Status epilepticus: a continuous seizure that lasts over 30 minutes, or two or more seizures without regaining consciousness in between any of them.]*

I'd suffered pains to my right temple and sharp jabs. As the days passed, it'd appeared that my seizures had changed. I hadn't lost awareness during most of the episodes and had been aware of what my body had done. The paralysis and shaking hadn't been typical of how the seizures had presented themselves at the beginning. As the neurons misfired, my left side responded. Paralyzed, my big toe would bend while the remaining digits stood at attention. The left fingers would spread apart as if readying themselves for the piano and curled downwards. They looked like talons from a bird of prey—an eagle or falcon preparing to grab its intended target as it swooped in for the kill. Preliminary results showed the seizures had been happening further back than expected. Beyond where the nine electrodes could detect them. I needed more holes. Back to the MRI, the needles, cage, and drill. Six more holes and tiny wires bored into my noggin, bringing the total to fifteen. Round two was a breeze, and I cracked jokes in the OR. I likened the drill to the old cartoon Woody Woodpecker—its metal shaft drilling holes into my skull like the woodpecker's beak digging into the bark of a tree.

To pass the time after my sister had left, I brought pre-moistened gloves and socks filled with peppermint and almond oil. Stretched out, hands and feet covered and listening to music was my Spa day at Foothills Chateau, as I called it. November's tracking calendar had filled up with notes from each day's activities: waves, seizures, Ativan and pain. Some days, my writing wasn't legible and made little sense.

*So. Here I sit surrounded by familiar strangers– individuals who look after me, treat me like family. They laugh and joke and hold my hand. They wipe my tears as my body rips apart. Foothills, my home away from the stress and worries that clouded my mind–Devon—my health–money–the future, and on, and on. No wonder I could seize and wave so easy back at home. All those thoughts had coiled around my brain, squeezed it–tightened–released and tightened again. It must've looked like a doggy balloon a clown had made, all twisted and bulging and ready to burst.*

By November 16th, I was off all meds except my Dilantin. On the mornings I awoke early, I'd stayed awake, recreating my version of sleep deprivation, hoping to have triggered a seizure.

**November 17, 2017, Journal entry**

*No action. I'd believed my body had deceived me and the doctors. Had I been wasting their time? It hadn't mattered how often I'd suffered through a seizure or how many pills I'd had to swallow, or how many doctors I'd seen, all the tests, and surgeries, it'd all led back to that moment. Why hadn't I'd produced enough seizures? Where'd all those waves and thunderstorms gone? Had my brain gone on holiday? It hadn't any problem until then inconveniencing my life, so why had it become silent? Stage-fright? Okay. So. You've had your fun, and it was time to stop. It's my life, and it's time you moved on— get back to the shadows where you'd sprung from and leave me the fuck alone.*

I confided in Dr. Young about my concerns–that I'd been wasting their time and maybe I'd been causing the seizures–that it'd been my fault. He assured me that epilepsy could change. That the brain could rewire itself and learn new pathways. He also stated that after the insertion of the wires, the brain could go dormant and wouldn't produce any seizures. I just had to be patient.

"Linda, you're having a seizure," Opal said, wandering into my room one day. I was on the phone and slow to react. I glanced at the screen, at the squiggly lines, brows furrowed, looking at her as if she were nuts. After hanging up, I sat watching the wavy lines move across the screen, unsure of or if they meant anything. That morning, I had awakened early with a wave. Full rising, tingly arms, powerful waves that surged and burned. My fingers were stiff and puffed up. Thus, began my second status epilepticus event. This time it'd lasted for eight hours. Just like the previous one, I'd lost awareness. The seizure started and had stopped and restarted. Apparently, the nurse had attempted to start a new IV, but had had to stop because I'd said it hurt. I'd had no recollection of it. They had made many phone calls to the neurologist for instructions. They had fed multiple doses of Ativan through the IV. Administering the dose straight into the bloodstream could react quicker than if given orally. The doctor even ordered a round of Dilantin, hoping it could work in tandem with the Ativan and could stop the attack. Eventually it had stopped in the early morning hours. I hadn't come to until almost noon. I'd been dopey, confused, battered and sore, and barely moved. It had taken up to three days for the drugs to leave my system.

Throughout my stay, I experienced multiple seizures. Some had begun with a wave, followed with stiffened legs and arms that wouldn't move no matter how hard I'd tried to raise them off of the bed. Once or twice an arm flopped up and down like a caught fish gasping for air. Another instance included the smell of burnt sawdust, similar to splicing through a damp log with a chainsaw. I'd heard music and thought someone was behind my bed. I'd talked to '*them*' about the song and how I couldn't recall the name. Another occurred where I'd felt a presence behind me leaving the bathroom, but no one was there.

It was Dr. O'Connor who'd delivered the results. The committee made up of epileptologists, neurologists and surgeons all agreed. Another trip into my wormhole to tunnel further back and remove more of the temporal lobe (the right posterior superior temporal gyrus). He'd showed most of the seizures I'd had were from the same section of the temporal lobe they'd removed last year. In addition, there'd been another area, the right insula. It was unknown if the insula had been the culprit or a by-product from the firing temporal lobe. The insula, surrounded by a dense highway of blood vessels, would be too risky to remove. If one or more vessels were severed, it could cause a stroke or brain damage. They would leave it alone.

*[Insula (or Insular cortex) allows us to feel pain and basic emotions and handles addictive behaviour, such as OCD.]*

Dr. Taylor, concerned with how much to remove from the temporal lobe without causing sensory issues, ordered a cortical brain stimulation test. Dr. Eastman would perform the exam.

"Don't worry Ms. McClure. This won't hurt: it'll tingle more than anything." They connected me to a device that'd sported a large black dial with white numbers printed all around it. A window with a red needle, a semicircle in black against a white background, rested above, protected by a clear plastic cover. It'd looked like it'd belonged back in the 1960s, when electric shock therapy was still a thing. As Dr. Eastman turned the dial up, he asked if I'd felt any pins and needles, and where. He'd tested the sensory areas of my face, arms, and legs–each time turning up the dial to gauge a response. At one point, I'd stated, "You look like you're enjoying this too much, Dr. Eastman. You're like the Nutty Professor!" I joked.

"Oh? That's good, because I am a nutty professor!" He laughed and pretended to crank the dial up all the way. Tired from the added stimuli, I'd lowered the head of my bed and slept until dinner.

It was then that I'd first heard about Psychogenic Non-Epileptic Seizures. I remember sitting on the bed, staring at Dr. O'Connor. His words hit me hard. He might as well have punched me in the gut. Told that I might have 'make-believe' seizures left me feeling guilty. As if I'd been lying the whole time and wasting theirs. The good news was there'd be no prescription. What I needed was therapy with a neuropsychologist, but there weren't any at home. Surprise surprise. What did we have? Not much. I had Dr. Edwards, thank God, and a failing medical system. The best we could do was bring Dr. Everly into the loop. She was a psychiatrist, a good one, and all I had available to me back in BC.

*[Psychogenic non-epileptic seizures (PNES) are paroxysmal episodes, often misdiagnosed as epileptic seizures. PNES are psychological (i.e., emotional, stress-related, trauma).]*

November 22nd: the probes had come out–I'd sported my Medusa Look for sixteen days–had fifteen holes drilled into my head. I couldn't wait to have a shower and wear my own clothes. I'd been living in pyjamas that'd fermented my sweat and body odour into a fragrance fit for a skunk. With the wires removed, I'd had a final CT scan, packed up my belongings and headed out. The flight back to BC was uneventful until I disembarked. Unsure of where to go and a little wobbly, I fought with my coat, missing the sleeve, tangling myself up as I tried to get my arm into it. A six-year-old would have managed better.

Back at home, sleeping in my bed did not stop the impulses firing within my battered head. Voices, odd sounds and conversations lost within the tangled neurons and anxious wavy sensations, the likes of which I experienced three years before, were constant. With no neuropsychologist available, my GP, Dr. Alisen, set out to get me in to see Dr. Everly. It took a few days before she could arrange something. Knowing my fragile mindset, Dr. Alisen kept me updated on her progress. Her persistence paid off, and scheduled an appointment for January 10, 2018.

Through Dr. Everly, I learned how productive my stay in the SMU had been. Sixteen seizures over 17 days, and only two were Psycho seizures (my name for them). I tried to keep tally in my journal, but had lost count. No wonder I felt as if I had run the Boston Marathon twice over. Relaxed on her couch, we discussed my moods and options for therapy. Leaning back in her chair, she would make the odd scribble, maintaining eye contact as often as possible. I mentioned the neuropsychiatrist BC Epilepsy had suggested, but the neuropsychiatrist worked with patients already established with a primary therapist. They'd create the treatment plan and left it to the primary therapist to implement it. I'd had no other option but to continue seeing Dr. Everly for as long as possible. But the program she worked under was just a filler between GP and long-term therapy and only provided so many visits.

# Chapter Thirteen

## **Surgery and a Storm on the Horizon**

*From January to February, my waves, the anxious, wavy sensations, continued in tandem with jabs of pain and memory issues. The tracking calendar became my 'journal' for the month, documenting the daily events as they happened in the notes section. I mentioned the light thingy was back in both eyes- started mid-February. Entries of strange sensations, my head feeling numb as if wrapped up in batten. Mixing and jumbling up my words. Ghost images, Waves, breaking out in cold sweats and awareness of consciousness sliding away in varying degrees. It was interesting to see a pattern emerge as my brain went through its cycles—how the waves fluctuated from day-to-day, week-to-week. One moment I'd be fine. The next, nausea would hit and send me reeling—plummeting and rising as if on a roller coaster. Sharp jabs of pain attacked my head. Wavey sensations started and stopped—the beginnings of a wave. Bouts of insomnia left me dopey throughout the day. As the surgery date approached, they'd increased from once or twice a week to everyday.*

My 2<sup>nd</sup> surgery was March 13, 2018, and coordinating my sibling's schedules with the surgeon had been a challenge. Planning this return trip to Calgary and seeking therapy overwhelmed me, and resulted in back-to-back seizures. It was the first time I had experienced such an event at home.

*\*\*March 2018—The wormhole's reopened\*\**

Margaret and I flew out on *March 11, 2018.* It was my fourth trip in the last year. I was much calmer than the first time. My hopes were high that this one would do the trick. That I would find some relief. Rebuild my life back to where it had been, or as close to it as possible. I wasn't nervous. The opposite, in fact—blasé. Another early morning. Sign in; wait over there, put on this gown. Lay down, close your eyes. And wait. MRI accomplished. Wheeled away to the corral. Doze off — last trip to the bathroom. Enter OR and strapped in place. IV inserted — oxygen mask in position. And we're off.

I woke in a much better state than last time. The pain didn't register as a 7.9 earthquake, instead, it was more like a tremor or aftershock. I was moving about soon after, which surprised the nurses. I felt good, considering they split my head open like a coconut. Scooped brain matter out like ice cream. One would think I had not had brain surgery as I ate, drank, and took myself to the washroom. Not drugged up on morphine or Percocet, I engaged in the goings-on around me. This time I wasn't the poor thing bundled up in blankets, head covered in ice packs too doped up to eat or drink. Margaret was ecstatic.

"You're doing so well we could be back home by the weekend. Wouldn't that be great?" She stated the next day.

I wasn't too sure about that, but what did I know? That night while asleep, my oxygen levels dropped. We don't know why. I was drinking and eating; there didn't seem to be a reason. Going home would be on hold until my levels increased. The surgical team popped in once or twice to check on my status. I needed to increase my food and water intake and move around more. Taking me to the bathroom and going for short walks.

My oxygen levels went back up and seemed to be fine; now it was up to me and how I was feeling as when I could leave.

"We can go home on Friday. Isn't that great? Let's get you packed up so we can skedaddle out of here." Margaret began gathering up things. Pulled clothes out for me to change into and checked cupboards and drawers.

As much as I wanted to go home, I didn't want to leave yet. My room, the nurses and doctors made me feel safe; and protected. I was a baby bird nestled in a cradle of comfort and warmth, cared for by those sympathetic to my needs. At home, I'm exposed to the elements and preyed upon by life's challenges alone in my fight for normalcy. I had no choice but to leave. Two days after my surgery, I was free to spread my wings. We booked the flight for the next day. Mom would have dinner with me and stay until Dev got home from work. No one wanted me left alone, "just in case." The flight was uneventful, as was the drive home and dinner. Mom headed out after Dev arrived with strict instructions that I was not to do any unpacking.

**The Clot**

All snuggled in pyjamas and housecoat; we sat watching TV. I remember the glass slipping from my left hand, spilling

217

its contents onto my lap. I sat for a moment, staring at my lap. The water pooled on my housecoat, soaking my pyjamas right through to the couch. I called out for Ativan and a towel— speech, slow and garbled. Devon took one look at me and sprung to his feet.

"You alright Mom?"

"y-e-s-th, y-u-m f-f-t-h-ine." The words sputtered as I struggled to push them out of my mouth.

"Mom, you're having a stroke. See, your mouth is drooping here, and you sound funny." He pointed to the left side of my mouth.

"y-u-m a-v-in-n a s-l-e-a-zur."

"No, it's a stroke. I'm calling 911." I tried to stop him, but the words were a jumbled mess. The sounds coming out were jibber-jabber, as if two mega-sized jawbreakers were in my cheeks. The paramedic arrived and crouched at my feet, assessing the situation. Checking my vitals and the pronounced weakness of my left side and drooping face, they determined I was having a stroke. I was adamant; it was a seizure. The words came out muddled, a string of nonsense; indistinguishable gobbledygook. If he understood my garble-talk, he ignored it. In his mind, I was stroking. At the hospital, I lay in what looked like a storeroom. In my fogged-up mind, I saw metal racking and discarded equipment—not an exam room. I struggled to speak. I hadn't taken my pills. The words weren't getting through—contained within the bubble surrounding my mind. Some found their way out and a faceless voice told me no medication until I saw the neurosurgeon — in case surgery was necessary. What? I can't go with no meds. I had brain surgery; I must take my pills. My brain is healing. I can't have seizures. It felt like the bubble was closing in, cutting off my oxygen supply. My words fought to get out—tell them they were wrong. But they didn't give in. Although I seized once more, nothing would happen until the morning after I transferred and saw the neurosurgeon. It was almost 5 pm the next day before I got my meds. I had gone without since 8 or 9 am Calgary time the day before. Two whole doses missed.

My bubble, still intact, produced a distorted view of my world. They moved me into a room and placed me onto a bed, but it wasn't until much later that I realized I had roommates. An elderly fellow laid across from me, hooked up to a tank. He had problems breathing, and he wore a mask unless he ate. Either the tank size was inefficient, or his lungs were of considerable size because the frequency of which they'd replaced the tanks was astounding. As each emptied, an alarm would sound—day or night. The constant beeping had gone unnoticed by my neighbour to the right. Unable to mumble more than a word or two, she had lain in a semi-conscious state letting her call bell to speak for her, and it too went off day and night. She and the last occupant had window seats overlooking the river. The poor lady at the far end was from out of town with no relatives close. She'd had back surgery and was in a lot of pain. She grumbled about no salt or ketchup and groused about the food. The neurosurgeon was the stereotypical absentminded scientist. He'd looked as if he'd just got out of bed—hair mussed and shuffling about like a sleepwalker. He told me I'd had a blood clot. *What?* He confirmed that I hadn't stroked. Well, I'd known that, but they hadn't listened to me. What he didn't know was if the clot had caused the seizure or the surgery had caused the clot. Regardless, I was to stay put until it'd dissolved. It would be a day or two or more. *Wonderful.*

Bored, I'd wanted to go home—I missed my bed, my food—my space. Although I was closer to home, my past experiences in hospital hadn't provided the calming atmosphere I'd felt in Foothills. My confidence in BC's medical system was tainted. To break up the days, I played nursemaid to my roomies. When I needed more water, I'd shuffle from bed to bed, gathered up jugs, filling each, and deposited them on table trays with a smile. And you're welcome. Nurses on our ward scuttled about answering call bells for meds and trips to toilets. Removing our meal trays had been at the bottom of their list. Staring at half-eaten scraps, cellophane wrappings, and empty creamers were far from appealing. Tired of waiting, I'd shifted my tray to the small counter at the door. Soon followed by my neighbour's dishes—piled one on top of another—they sat awaiting removal. These minor tasks got me up and moving, and as I'd wandered up and down in between the beds. Standing at the window, I'd had the view of the flowing river outside pushing the logs downstream as they'd bob along in the steady current. The serenity of witnessing mother nature at work had soothed me—it was a balm to my turbulent thoughts.

During the week's stay, I endured another seizure milder than the last two. Three events since my surgery two weeks before concerned me. At night, I'd curled up in a ball with the blanket covering my mouth and sobbed. I'd convinced myself the operation had failed. I would write in my journal, the tears splashing on the page. The blood clot compounded the issue and brought back memories of how my dad had died. Like my neighbour next to me, he'd had a brain aneurysm that ruptured, the damage killing him. And he wasn't the only family member that succumbed to their brain. My little niece's candle snuffed out at twenty-two months, an issue with blood vessels or some such thing. I'd wonder if that, too, will be my fate. My brain damaged beyond repair. That it would short circuit and explode, cutting off power to my body, the life source extinguished. I knew it was irrational, not possible that I'd face the same outcome, and I'd tried my best to ignore those thoughts. The month hadn't been easy, and to dispel the doom and gloom of a dismal future had seemed impossible. I'd felt isolated and alone, trapped within a mind bent on destruction. Afraid to leave and yet couldn't wait to get home. Just as my body had been battling a faceless attacker, my emotional state had spun out of control. From fear—to boredom—eager to leave, but afraid to go–frustrated–worried–sad. I'd been a muddled up–disjointed; a scrambled mess.

On March 23rd, they discharged me. The blood clot had dispelled and no further seizures occurred. That night I finally slept in my bed, a week later than planned.

**April 5, 2018—Back to the neurosurgeon**

"Hello, Ms. McClure. How're you feeling? Any headaches, seizures?" Dr. Sam waved at a stool next to his desk for me to sit on and sat down. He shuffled through my chart.

His desktop was littered with charts, medical books, newspapers, pens, and notepads.

"No, no headaches, other than my normal. From my surgeries and the nerve pains. No seizures either since you saw me in hospital." I hadn't known what to expect from this visit. Only came for a follow-up from the clot. I wouldn't see him again and wasn't sure why I had to come to begin with. In his professional opinion, the surgery had caused the blood clot. The seizure, an unfortunate event. He couldn't do anything for me and warned I could see an increase in seizures because of the scarring.

"You should follow up with your neurologist." His only recommendation. My forty-five-minute drive had resulted in a two-minute visit that could've happened at the hospital before he'd discharged me, or by phone. Knowing what I know now, my chances of seizure freedom were zero — continuing with anticonvulsants a sure thing. The odds were against me right from the start. Lady Luck had left the building.

*\*\*\*The calm before the storm\*\*\**

I saw Dr. Edwards the day after the neurosurgeon. He hadn't confirmed or denied his prediction of further seizures. He'd explained that the blood clot bled into the surgical cavity. There was no damage done to the brain. He, too, believed the surgery caused the clot. Whether flying home so soon afterwards had contributed to the seizure was unknown, but it hadn't caused it, so I wasn't to fret about it. We'd discussed the pains I still experienced, and my use of the Percocet. I tried not to rely on it and used Tylenol to keep a lid on it. He'd mentioned switching up my meds.

"I want to remove the Topamax and the Dilantin and start you on Vimpat. You'd get better long-term control by moving to the newer drug." He'd said. I'd been on Dilantin since the start. It wasn't the best drug for a woman of my age, as it contributed to bone loss and promoted hair growth in all the wrong places. But it'd been too soon to start the plan. The added complication of the blood clot and only a month out from surgery would've put me in a tailspin. June or July would be soon enough.

The following week I saw Dr. Everly. It'd been my third doctor's appointment in eleven days. I brought her up to speed on my adventures over the last month. She couldn't believe what I'd been through and pressed me about writing a book. She sat reclined in her chair, her eyes locked on mine.

"Your story is unique and astounding. The challenges you've faced would've crumbled anyone else. You need to share your experiences. I'll be interested to see how it all plays out."

I nodded, staring at the floor, hands clasped, a weight on my shoulders heavier than the couch I'd sat upon. We chatted about my feelings and emotional state of mind and how to move forward.

"Sorry to say this, Linda. But I'm afraid I've pushed the boundaries of the Rapid Access Program, and I won't be able to see you again without a new referral." They designed the Rapid Access Program as a starting point for patients with mental health issues. It was and is a temporary fix for the deficiencies within the health system. Easy access to mental health professionals didn't exist. The Rapid Access Program granted a limited amount of appointments to a psychiatrist. It was never the intention to take the place of ongoing therapy. For that, you had to pay. Because of the limitations she had to cut me loose to fight the fears and anxieties alone. Not the doctor's fault. It was the medical system. And no matter how much support I'd received from others, I was in this nightmare by myself.

A phone appointment with my epileptologist, Dr. Young, was two weeks later to check in and see how things were since my surgery. I sat at the dining room table with papers spread out around me nibbling on some carrots, cheese, and almonds, as I watched the leaves swaying on the trees and butterflies and bees flitted about in search of food. My notes weren't finished but I could reference the more prominent calendar entries for April.

*April 8 Wave full rising one min*

*April 10 mumbling? — ghost image — wavey cold sweat or hot flash?*

*April 14: fuzzy, confused, 1st thing—tingling on cheeks — lightheaded — rising three to four minutes. Wave.*

*April 21 Wave churning — 'off' feeling — nerves tingly lasted a min-tired after wavey at bed*

*April 22 looked like room turning — lightheaded — unsteady, weak, tired, woozy,*

*April 23 A wave or a strong Anxious Wavey Feeling woke me — took a bit to focus and wake up*

*April 24 lightheaded at one point — felt like passing out for a min—pains on and off*

*Note: On April 10th when filling pill box-started putting Dilantin in the AM slot vs PM didn't clue in until week was just about filled (I start with the AM dose then move to PM, if I didn't notice I may have double dosed myself)*

*April Totals: Wave: 6 Wavey: 8 Wavey/Anxious: 11 Ghost Images: 12 Seizures: 2? Ativan: 0*

I mentioned the blood clot and Dr. Edwards's plans for my medication changes. Dr. Young concurred with Dr. Edwards's plan, and we scheduled my six-month follow-up for August 1st. Three weeks after my call with Dr. Young was my surgical follow up with Dr. Taylor. They had arranged it for him to call between 2-4 pm. When my phone rang at 7:30 am, I was unprepared. I'd been awake, tossing and turning, plumping up pillows to cradle my head to lull me back to sleep. But it didn't work. Exasperated, I'd pushed the blankets out of my way. My feet touched the floor seconds before he'd called. Groggy with sleep, my mind couldn't focus. All the notes were on my laptop that'd sat idle on the desk. He called in between patients and had little time. Our conversation lasted three minutes, and it was a bust. I stared at the crafted notes saved on my laptop. That had been useless. I asked if maybe I flew home too soon. Did the surgery cause the clot? He answered no to both. It wasn't until afterwards when I reviewed my notes, I hadn't asked about recovery time. How long before I could resume my workouts? Was there any damage caused by the clot and the seizures? The call was a complete waste of his time. Although it wasn't my fault, I felt guilty.

Looking back at all my notes and calendars now amazes me how much activity occurred during those months. With careful precision, I'd track the day-to-day events in my notebook, starting another as the pages filled up, and added them to the pile of symptoms and observations. The first days of each month found me hunched over my desk, notebook at the ready, pen poised, deciphering, editing, and transferring the details to my calendar document on Word. I'd thumb through pages covering a month's worth of activity; how often each wave, ghost image, wavey sensation occurred. Seeing it laid out on one page, each box representing a day, brought it to life. Tallying them up made it worse. After two surgeries and the twenty-one pills per day, things hadn't changed much. Well, it had, but only to the point of remaining conscious until the Ativan knocked me out. I no longer had the awful odours, and the waves weren't as often. Back in 2015, I'd had fifty in one month—or was it 2016? May had turned out better than April. My brain was healing, and I'd felt positive about the future — that this was the one that did it. Life had looked good. My spirits had lifted, and I smiled and laughed more—freedom was just around the corner. Or so I thought.

*\*\*Black Clouds Gather—June 2018\*\**

For the first time since I'd purchased my townhouse back in 2009, I had an infestation of carpenter ants. Different from black ants, their bodies are more inline with humans. Small head and large behinds. I first noticed them in the living room. Crawling along windowsills, the carpet, around the patio door, and into the kitchen. Their mission: rotten, wet wood—a mecca for hungry destroyers. Like an infantry, they fanned out, seeking sustenance, going from room to room, displaying no fear of the cat. Ant baits and sprays were useless. An exterminator was necessary to eradicate the pests, and we had to vacate the premises, yard included, for eight hours. It meant we had to remove our indoor cat to the great outdoors and hope he didn't escape. I was no longer the planner and organizer I'd been before, and it placed a tremendous amount of stress upon my feeble mind. No harness was big enough for our eighteen-pound of lard. He couldn't stay in his crate for eight hours without a litter box. Lucky for us, our neighbour was going away and had offered us the shelter of her home, cat included. Problem solved.

*\*\*June 2, 2018 calendar entry\*\**

*I'm not one hundred percent sure, but believe I saw someone walking by my kitchen window, or the definite shape of a human body. Standing off to the side, looking at my phone and swiping away silly notifications from the screen I thought I saw movement. I looked up and thought I saw someone walking. I looked out the window and opened my front door, but didn't see anybody. I could have missed them, or I'm losing my mind.*

*\*\*June 30, 2018 note\*\**

*Went to take evening pills and discovered my PM slots in my pillbox were all screwed up. Saturday to Tuesday was missing Clobazam Sunday had doubled the Dilantin dose.*

I refused to let the mix-up deter my desire for independence. Taking these pills was now a part of my daily routine I had to manage. I required support in so many areas of my life and was determined to control this. Despite the added stressors, I'd made it through the month unscathed. Yes, I'd had seizures, and needed Ativan, and experienced other events which had become my norm, but it could've been worse. It could've been like July.

My brief visit with Dr. Edwards at the end of June had set the plan in motion for shifting me from the Topiramate and Dilantin over to Lacosamide (aka Vimpat). I'd start by adding it in and then wean off the Topiramate and Dilantin. The new drug wasn't cheap — a few hundred dollars for a meagre amount. The kitchen counter had looked like a shelf in a drugstore. Five or six bottles, a box or two, and my pillbox had taken over one corner.

*\*\*July 2018, calendar entries\*\**

*July 3, 2018, seizure at mall.*

*July 4, 2018 day one of Lacosamide-bit of head rush wave-type seizure feeling after taking the first dose.*

*July 5, 2018–head rush etc. not as bad today.*

*July 8, 2018 thought I heard a 'beep' during the night.*

*July 10, 2018 anxious wavey feeling dazed staring at tv not moving — body heavy — hands tingly, about 10 min. Weak after.*

*July 11,2018 Lacosamide at one hundred and fifty milligrams. Ghost images. Felt 'high' 'drunk' — unsteady at first when out for a walk. Balance has been more of an issue. 'Things' crawling on me and prickly again.*

*July 12, 2018 anxious wavey feeling ghost images, strong wavey period flushed <five minutes dopey/woozy itchy lower legs,*

*July 13, 2018 ghost images seizure. Prickly feeling on r-shin twice.*

After the first week of July, I was up to six meds and felt worse than I had in ages. I trudged about, moving from floor to floor out of need. My bed and shower were up on the third. I scrounged for food in the kitchen and often ate straight from the pantry or fridge. When necessary, I ventured down to the basement to wash clothes stale from body sweat and covered in cat hair. As the days ticked by, I became concerned. I'd had two seizures in ten days, was dopey, wavy and out of sorts. In desperation, I emailed Dr. Edwards.

*From: Linda McClure*
*Sent: July 13, 2018 9:28 PM*
*To: Dr. Edwards*
*Subject: Question for Dr. Edwards re Lacosamide*

*Happy Friday!*

*Sorry to bother you but wanted to ask you:*

*Is there a possibility the Lacosamide doesn't "play nice" with my other medications and it neutralizes the effectiveness of them?*

*Just curious, as I'm on 6 AEDs and still having seizures, so was looking to you for your infinite wisdom.*

*Since starting Lacosamide on July 4th, I believe I've had 2 seizures. The last one being today, July 13th.*

*Following a ½ hour nap, I woke feeling dazed out of it.*

*—toes right side tingled (pins and needles) followed by entire leg*

*—body felt heavy- very hard to move-it was possible, but difficult. Right side of head all prickly like a nerve thing-pulsating.*

*—Followed by prickly feeling in right shin again.*

*—Speech delayed and slow to respond. As per Annie(on phone)*

*—lasted approx.15-20min total.*

*— Lacosamide: I'm taking 150mg twice a day. Increasing to 200mg on Wed July 18th.*

*— I have noticed balance issues, drowsiness and lack of energy*

*—a significant increase in focusing on reading and/or writing (nodding off after reading for short periods)*

*— I found the increase from 100mg to 150mg caused an excessive 'high' effect for the first few days.*

*— The itchiness and prickly sensations I spoke of back on June 29th still come and go.*

*That's all I have for now. Have a wonderful weekend!*

*Sincerely,*


Linda


Disturbed that the Vimpat had made no difference and had made things worse, I emailed Dr. Edwards again three days later.

**Sent:** *July 16, 2018 5:31 PM*

**To:** *Dr. Edwards*

**Subject:** *McClure, Linda–SEIZURE UPDATE*

*Good Afternoon, Dr. Edwards*

*Further to my email from Friday, July 13th, I wanted to let you know that I had a 2nd seizure on Sunday, July 15th while out shopping with Devon in Walmart.*

*· I had some sharp pains & jabs prior to us leaving and took an Extra Strength Advil.*

*· Unsure how long we'd been shopping prior to start of Seizure.*

*· Same "washing over" sensation felt as in your office on June 29th, but not as intense.*

*· Could see Dev and hear him, but unable to respond at first and then very limited.*

*· Didn't want to take Ativan.*

*· It subsided in about 5 minutes, maybe longer.*

· *Devon's observation: I stood there unable to move and "zoned out." Speech slow/slurred.*

· *Tired and moving slow afterwards, but paid for our stuff, got a cab and went home.*

· *Slept for an hour.*

· *Found a note on phone from 11:12 am stating "felt WAVEY." No memory of writing it.*

· *Since my surgery on March 13th, I've had 10 Seizures now.*

· *I'm thinking this surgery, combined with the blood clot, made things worse. Prior to either of my surgeries, only my Waves occurred with the same level of frequency in such a short time.*

· *Do you think this is just a short-term thing that will settle down as my brain heals more?*

· *It's been 4 months since the surgery and I know the brain needs time and with the added complication I had, it will need even more.*

· *What about the changes to my medications?*

*· Will we be looking to hold off removing anything for a bit?*

*· I started the Lacosamide on July 4th, increased dose to 150mg on July 11th, then had a seizure on July 13th & 15th.*

*· Any thoughts on this? Are you able to talk me off of the ledge, so to speak?*

*Thank you for your time.*

*Sincerely,*


Linda


When I hadn't received a reply, I called the office. Angela informed me he was away—out of the country and couldn't be reached. He was due back mid-August, a whole month away, and would address my concerns once back in the office. I had to persevere until then or discuss it with Dr. Young when I saw him on *August 1, 2018.*

July 21st, I had my next seizure. It'd happened after I'd taken my evening pills at 8:30 pm. My body felt heavy and I could hardly move. I sat staring at the TV for a bit. I became woozy, breathing hard at one point and my eyes kept closing like at the eye doctors when he uses that big thing over your eyes and flips the lens, switching eyes. The right one goes black while testing the left. Flip–flop–flip–flop. My head and body heavy, tired. Slowly I managed to move my legs–they were so weak I couldn't stand. It passed after ten to fifteen minutes, but the weakness lasted a bit longer. By the time I'd recuperated, it'd been 9:30pm before I'd crawled to bed.


Five days later, I was in the shower when I felt funny. My head didn't feel quite right. I stood and stared at the shower wall. I had no clue how long I'd been standing there when my breathing became laboured and my chest heavy. My vision became narrowed, edged in black–the shower was closing in, darkening my surroundings. I remember calling out to Dev, but it'd been more like grunts. I wasn't shaking and my limbs could move, but I was weak. I had to lean against the cold tile of the shower. I'd thrown items from the corner caddy onto the floor. A shampoo bottle, soap, and a hairbrush. I was afraid to get out by myself. We had a deep soaker tub and there had been no counter or ledge outside to grab onto. Eventually, Dev came and helped me out. He held my arms to steady me, sat me on the edge of the tub, and wrapped me in a towel. Dressed in my housecoat and seated upon my bed, he gave me an Ativan. The entire experience had exhausted me, shaken me up. I recall lying down curled into a ball, wanting to throw up.

*\*\*August 1, 2018–In person follow-up with Dr. Young*

*Foothills Hospital–Calgary\*\**

We'd flown out on July 31 and flew back home the next day after we'd seen Dr. Young at 11 am.

The reception handed me forms for completion before my appointment. I hadn't completed them when the receptionist escorted Dev and me to a small office. The room was the basic sterile white box with linoleum floor, posters of brains and the neural highway connecting the byways and side streets. We'd tried our best to answer the remaining questions, but still hadn't finished when Dr. Young arrived.

"Hello Linda, thanks for coming in. How was your flight? Did you arrive today or yesterday?" He breezed into the room, swinging the door behind him. It made a soft thud as the latch clicked into place. The thick chart under his arm made more noise as it'd hit the desk with a loud thump.

"Oh, Dr. Young, this is my son Devon. I don't believe you've met him before."

"Hi," Dev held out his hand to shake his.

"It's nice to meet you. Are you taking good care of your mother?" He'd smiled and turned to flip through the mounds of paper next to him.

"Have you finished with those?" He reached for the forms that laid on the desk in front of me—still unfinished.

"Uh, no, I was having a hard time understanding some questions and didn't know how to answer them." I slid the sheets over, thinking he'd read what I'd put and file them away. After looking them over, he'd turned them around so I could see them right side up. He looked from me to Dev and back again. His face was like stone. He pointed at the first question and had slid his index finger down the page.

"Linda, these aren't hard questions. Read them and pick the best option. Come on; you can do it." Hesitantly, I pulled them closer, had leaned forward and scanned the page before stopping at the first one. Pointing at it, I'd said.

"I'm not sure how to answer this. Sometimes I feel this way, but not always. It varies. I don't know which one to pick."

"Linda, it's easy. Go with your gut. The answer doesn't have to be concise. You select the one which is closest to what is going on." Sitting back, he'd crossed his arms and legs, frustrated, almost annoyed.

"Sir, she's right. This question makes little sense. It's not worded right." Dev turned the page back to him, pointing to the wording.

Uncrossing his limbs, Dr. Young leaned forward and read the page. "Hmm. You're right. How did that happen? Good catch, I must get this fixed."

"Oh, and here too isn't correct." Dr. Young glanced over it a second time.

"Would you like a job?" His joke eased the tension that had built within me.

I was nervous, couldn't stop myself from fidgeting. I rubbed my hand down my thigh as if to remove something that hadn't been there. His attention turned back to me as he'd laid the paper down.

"Dr. Edwards advised me you've added the Vimpat and are preparing to reduce your other medications. I'm going to suggest we start with the Topiramate and then go from there." He grabbed a blank sheet of paper and wrote out the weaning schedule I'd had to follow. It'd be a gradual process. My dosage was to reduce weekly.

*[Antiseizure medications can not just be stopped without dire circumstances. To just stop the constant flow suddenly could cause severe side effects, one of them being seizures.]*

He spoke aloud as he wrote, glanced up as he moved from week to week to be sure I'd understood the instructions. When he'd paused, I piped up.

"Dr. Edwards was looking at removing the Dilantin too."

"I concur. That leaves you with Lamotrigine, Clobazam, and Gabapentin. Which of these do you hate the most?" He pushed aside the paper he'd been working on and grabbed a fresh sheet.

"Clobazam," I stated. "It makes me dopey. I've never liked it from the start." My nose wrinkled as the name had left my mouth.

"Ok. We'll do that one next after the Topiramate." His writing was pointed and quick. Accustomed to making quick decisions and getting them down on paper at high velocity, he'd wasted no time scribbling the schedule to wean me off the hated drug. His task done, he relaxed back into his chair, crossed his legs, and made himself comfortable and stared at me. I felt uncomfortable. I had been about to speak when he uncrossed his arms, leaned his elbows on the desk and steepled his fingers.

"You know, you're a mystery, Ms. McClure. We don't know what to do about you. Your epilepsy is a challenge. It's acting progressive, and we don't know why. You're an enigma. But don't worry; we'll sort this out." Letting that sink in, he slid my instructions closer to me, while pulling the tomb that was my chart to him, and flicked open the top. "Do you have questions?"

Glancing at Devon, who sat head down reading his notes, I replied, "Um, yes. My Ativan. I'm getting low, and they've cracked down on doctors prescribing it. Could you write me a prescription and I'll fill it here before I go home?" I fiddled with the pages in front of me and shifted my eyes to his. He answered as he wrote my prescription on a pad that'd appeared out of his suit jacket? A sleeve?

"Yes, but try not to use it too much. Only when you're in a full-blown seizure. Not these waves and such." He pointed to the Wavy, Anxious/Wavy, and Ghost Images noted in my summary. I nodded and added it to my pile. With that, he rose, came around the desk, and stopped beside my chair. Cupping the right side of my head, he said, "Take care of yourself." His voice was soft, filled with empathy, his eyes had been gentle and kind. Before I could respond, he slipped out, leaving the door ajar.

Down to the main entrance, out the sliding doors, we climbed into the first available cab and made our way to the airport.

*[It'd taken a seizure, my epilepsy diagnosis, and two surgeries before I'd ever felt helpless. But it wasn't until the summer and fall of 2018 that I lost control. It'd been like falling without a parachute or a safety net below the tightrope. My best laid plans cast aside and all my backups disappeared— vanished. The chaos and turmoil within me had gone wild– untamed–intractable. To have regained the life I'd had was as fruitless as grabbing hold of a cloud. The disease was in the driver's seat — me, an unwilling passenger, along for a ride to hell and beyond.]*

# Chapter Fourteen

## *\*\* Black Clouds Fill the Sky\*\**

As soon as we got back home, I filled my prescription for the Topamax weaning and had it placed in blister packs. I'd already had mishaps before when I filled my pillbox and I'd forgotten to take them, or had double dosed myself. It'd be safer to prepackage them while we reduced the dosage. By the end of that first week, I reached the full dose of Vimpat. As the Vimpat had increased, the Topamax had reduced as Dr. Young prescribed. And yet, I still experienced difficulties. I blamed the Vimpat. I suspected it hadn't played nice to my other drugs, and the waves and seizure activity continued.

*August 17, 2018—My world spins out of control*

How it started is a blur. I was in the kitchen when I became disoriented, my world tilted and swayed like an empty swing in a breeze. I called out to Devon, my speech a mumbled, garbled mess as I fought to get the words out. I grasped the counter as my body weakened—fingers curled under the edge to keep me from falling to the floor. A chair appeared, and Devon had me sit. As it escalated, he'd placed an Ativan in my slackened mouth. It'd appeared it would stop, but then another had circled back. It hadn't wanted to let go. The seizures wouldn't stop and I went into status epilepticus and he called 911. I have a vague memory of the ambulance. Or it was a scene replayed from many times before. I remember the emergency entrance and waiting for the triage nurse. But if I'd had a scan, there's no memory of it. I ended up across from the nursing station, with the drapes closed on either side, but remained open on their end so they could monitor me. I'd continued to seize as nurses, doctors, and orderlies passed by, unaware of the woman that twitched on her bed. Eventually, a doctor came by with the results of my scan.

"There's a hole in your head there between your brows," he'd said and pointed to the space at the top of my nose. "And there's air in it." Then he'd moved on. *Was he serious?*

I stared at his back as he'd strode away, leaving me there stunned, frightened, and worried. I tried to convince myself he'd worked too many hours and couldn't see straight. The overcrowded emergency room was not the ideal place to monitor me. The nurses scurried in and around the beds, passed by me without a glance. They were too busy checking blood pressures, handing out pain killers, and changing IVs to notice a woman that'd tried to get their attention as she seized, unable to utter a sound. My voice box no longer worked, and I suffered in silence–the seizures hadn't stopped. I needed the bathroom, had to pee so badly my teeth were floating. I lost the call button; it slipped down the side of the bed–the cord no longer within my reach. My voice box jammed, and the nurses occupied elsewhere. An IV, blood pressure cuff, stickers with cables attached to my chest to monitor my heart made it impossible to get up unaided. With all the cords and wires attached to me, it appeared as though I was strapped to the bed. If it hadn't been for Michael, I'd have wet the bed. He was young for a nurse, had dark curly hair and big brown eyes. He saw me from the nurses' station as I tried to flag someone down to assist me.

"Hi there. Are you needing some help? What can I do? What do ya need?" Nurse Michael smiled at me as he checked my IV.

"Yes, thank you. Yes, please. I need to go to the bathroom. Like, really bad. I need help to get disconnected."

In short order, Michael had released me and escorted me to and from the washroom. Throughout his shift, he made a point of checking on me. He made sure I had plenty of water and disentangled me when I'd needed to relieve myself. He'd been a blessing and I don't know how'd I'd have managed that night without him.


It was after dinner before Margaret had arrived. She popped by to see how I was doing and to give me a hug. By then, a new doctor had come on shift. Dr. Chung. After he reviewed my scan, he determined that with the structural changes from my prior surgeries and the addition of thirteen holes from the depth probes had confused the previous doctor. I relaxed into the pillows, relieved there was no hole and no more air than there should've been, if any. As he inquired of how'd I'd landed in the emergency and what'd transpired since, another seizure occurred. I could see and hear him. My body twitched back and forth. I watched the expressions on his face change and could hear him speak, but as before, I had no voice. I strained to get words out but nothing came forth, not even a croak or a squeak. I'd become mute. My thoughts were shut away in my head–struggling to be heard. When it abated, he pulled my sister aside. They discussed my situation, and he expressed his reluctance to release me to my sister. When he'd left, Margaret told me his concerns, how the seizures had continued despite their efforts and that the neurologist scheduled for that day hadn't returned his call and Dr. Edwards hadn't returned. Margaret said they'd both agreed I couldn't stay in the emergency, but I couldn't go home. The only solution had been to admit me.

"I don't know when they'll move you. It all depends on when a bed becomes available. I'm going to head home, get some sleep, and come back tomorrow and check on you. Okay?" Her hand had been rubbing my back and squeezing the back of my neck to release some tension as she spoke. It had been calming, and I became sleepy. "You're going to be okay. Dr. Chung will look after you, alright?" All I could manage was a slight dip of my head in acknowledgement, and even that had been a struggle as the energy had dissipated, leaving me lifeless. It was almost midnight before they transported me up to the second floor. The next morning I awakened to a sun-filled room with a view of Mount Baker. But I hadn't cared. All I wanted was for the seizures to stop so I could go home.

### ***The Nightmare Begins***

My seizure frequency hadn't decreased; it ramped up to three or four *per day*. Dr. Chung had continued trying to reach Dr. Edwards for his help to defuse the attacks on my body. He was still out of the country. The hospital didn't have a neurological department. The neurologists from throughout the city rotated. Whoever had been on call was overloaded and ran off their feet. I never saw one. I spent a week in the hospital tormented and scared, afraid the seizures wouldn't stop. I felt alone and abandon–that there wasn't anyone who could've helped me. The nurses couldn't manage a patient with multiple seizures, they hadn't encountered a case such as mine. Not used to administering the Ativan at the frequency I required, they fumbled to prepare the needle to inject into my IV.

During my spells, I could see and hear, but couldn't speak. The seizures were long, lasting twenty minutes on average. It was *frightening* to feel my body not responding–to be aware of every twitch, jerk, and the muscles contracted, unable to move. My seizures had always been long, and these were no exception, except I experienced the sensations as they happened and couldn't do anything to stop them. Knowing what was going on and not able to communicate was more traumatic than losing consciousness and coming to in a hospital doped up on drugs. I almost felt sorry for the nurses and doctors–their own frustrations of not being able to ease my plight. That went away when one had tried pushing a thermometer into my mouth as I seized. Then later another had me face-planted into the mattress and had not tried to turn me over. Slumped in an awkward position, my mouth pressed to the sheet, I could only mumble — couldn't turn over. Breathing had been difficult with both mouth and nose blocked. Thank God my mother was there visiting.

"She *can't breathe*. Turn her over. *Hurry.*" She reached out, leaning forward from her chair tucked out of the way by the window. It was a full minute before Mom's words sunk in. Leaning over, the nurse grabbed my shoulder and, straining, rolled me over. Freed from my prison, my eyes wild, shifted about like an animal sensing danger, my stomach churned the panic abating. With fresh air in my lungs, I focused on calming the rapid beat of my heart–reducing the pressure of blood that rushed through my veins. I couldn't help but wonder: What *if* Mom hadn't been there? Would I have died? Her presence had been a relief.

"It's ok. You're alright now. It's over. Lay back and get some rest. I'm going to get a sandwich and something to drink.

I'll be right back. Ok?" She hugged me, patted my back, stroked my hair, and kissed my forehead. Anyone that glanced in would've seen a mother consoling her child as if she'd fallen off her bike and had skinned knees and elbows. A casual observer would've had no clue what had just transpired; would've assumed all was ok.

*From: Linda McClure*
*Sent: August 21, 2018 2:59PM*
*To: Dr. Edwards*
*Subject: McClure Linda–Status Seizure events*

*Hi Dr. Edwards*

*Dr. Chung admitted me into the Community Hospital after being brought into the emergency on Fri, August 17th, and is reluctant to discharge me until after speaking with you and Dr. Young. He's left phone messages for both of you and has left me on bed arrest until he feels comfortable letting me go home.*

*I've had an additional 5 seizures since then that I'm aware of. Dr. Chung's concern is sending me home when I spend a lot of time by myself.*

*If you can please find time to come discuss your pain in the ass patient's case with him or call him, I would appreciate it.*

*Sincerely,*

*Linda McClure*

*Ps. I'm to start week 3 of my Topamax weaning schedule tomorrow.*

# Chapter Fifteen

## **Hello? Can Anybody Help Me?**

My seizures hadn't improved, and Dr. Edwards was still away. Phone calls to his office and cell phone went unanswered, and the email I'd sent, begging for his help, floated in cyberspace. Despite Dr. Chung's efforts, I did not feel safe. And needed reinforcements. I resorted to calling Dr. Young and left him a message explaining my dilemma.

"Ms. McClure? What's going on? Tell me everything." Dr. Young returned my call within hours. I explained my situation. The words spewed out faster than running water picking up speed as the emotions poured forth. My volume increased as I recounted each event, and I didn't care who heard me. I told him about the Status epilepticus—the ongoing seizures—having not seen a neurologist and that Dr. Edwards had been away and wasn't returning phone messages or emails.

"Is it possible the Vimpat isn't helping? Like, could it be causing the seizures?" I laid on my side, faced away from the door, with my notebook on the bed in front of me.

"Yes, it's possible. You're still weaning off the Topiramate, yes?" I opened the drawer of my side table and pulled the blister packs out; a big grin planted on my face when I replied, "Yes. I'm driving the nurses nuts. I'm insisting on using my blister packs."

"Okay, but we should change that up a bit."

"Okay." I pulled my notebook closer, pen ready to jot down his instructions.

"We will keep the Topamax at 100 milligrams twice a day for now and continue reducing the Lacosamide to 100 milligrams in the morning and leave the evening dose at the 200 milligrams for the next week. If the Lacosamide caused the increase of seizure activity, reducing the dose will confirm it."

"Ok. Dr. Young? Can Dr. Chung call you? To get your advice?" I asked.

"Yes, definitely. You've got my number. Dr. Chung? Is it?"

"Yes, I do and, yes, Dr. Chung is the doctor."

"It's ok, Ms. McClure; we'll get this sorted out. Try to relax if you can. Take care." And he hung up.

He was my only lifeline, the only hope I had to get through. I felt better. It helped to have spoken with him. I didn't feel so alone and terrified afterwards. My tears hit the pages of my notebook—splashing onto the words written there. I put it and the blister packs away and rolled onto my back, pulled the blanket up around my shoulders and fell asleep.

Shift change. I was now in the hands of a third doctor, Dr. Johns. I'd had to relive the previous 24 hours filling in the details not covered in the few scribbled notes jotted down in haste by her two predecessors. *Oh, why hadn't Dr. Edwards called back? Why didn't he respond to my email?* I said to myself a hundred times. Tears of worry and dread broke through the wall I'd built to contain my fears. I kept asking myself: What's going to happen to me? At night, I dreamt I was drowning: my feet tied together with bricks at the end of a rope that dragged me under the ground. I'd awake feeling trapped, gasping for air and clawing at liquid dirt, trying to reach the top only to slide further back. In my dream, the enemy was winning as it drew me down deeper into the shadows whence it came. Come daylight, it continued, it hadn't been a dream. It had been real.

The situation still hadn't improved from when I'd last spoken to Dr. Young, and I became desperate and had left another message begging him to call.

"From where I stand, and I don't know all the details being here in Calgary, we should get you hooked up on EEG. You have two options. You can go to Victory Regional or Sullivan District. Which one do you pick?" I could tell we had frustrated him. Not because I'd called him, but that I'd had to call.

"Sullivan. Dr. Edwards runs a monitoring room there." I'd told him. I'd seen no reason in going to Victory Regional when I'd never been before, and by going to Sullivan, Dr. Edwards would be sure to get the results. It'd seemed like a good idea; in the moment. Looking back, it would've made more sense to have gone to Victory, where I would've been with doctors more familiar with cases such as mine. Could've, should've, would've as the saying goes. The old saying hindsight is twenty-twenty runs through my mind even today.

"So, Sullivan it is. We'll sort this out. Don't worry. Take care, Ms. McClure."

August 23, 2018, I received an email from Dr. Edwards's office manager, Angela. She wanted to book my next appointment and had assumed they had discharged me and I was back at home. I replied updating her of my predicament.

*Hi Angela,*

*I wish I could say I was back at home, but that is not the case.*

*I've continued experiencing 1-2 seizures/day, and lasting on average about 15-20 minutes. I believe Dr. Edwards is still away and not up-to-date with the situation. I'm waiting for transfer to Sullivan District Hospital, which should hopefully be over the next few days. My last conversation with Dr. Young was to consider transferring myself to either Victory Regional or Sullivan District in order to have access to a neurologist round the clock. And staff more familiar and experienced with my condition. I would hope to be home by September 5th, so could definitely take the appointment time, no problem. If any changes, I will let you know.*

Dr. Johns had arranged for my transfer to Sullivan for the next day. I felt better with the change in venue. The tension within my body had loosened–my teeth no longer clenched, had relaxed, reducing the pressure on the jaw, and my shoulders slumped down to their natural position below my earlobes. I'd be back to where I'd first met Dr. Edwards and be under the care of doctors and nurses more experienced with seizures. By then I'd been in the hospital for a week–arrived on August 17th and then shipped off to Sullivan on August 24th. I'd spent so many hours drugged up on Ativan that my memories of those seven days are limited. But what I hadn't realized was those experiences had been miniscule compared to what came after. I had no help from the staff to pack up my belongings. My friend Annie, who popped by to visit, took charge and loaded up my stuff in the drawstring bags the hospital had provided. She pulled clothes from the cupboard, the toothpaste, brush, and miscellaneous toiletries, the puzzle books and blister packs from the side table drawers. She'd just finished when the transport vehicle arrived.

"Thanks so much, Annie. I couldn't have managed without you. Love ya!" Loaded up on the stretcher, the paramedics had wheeled me down the hall and into the elevator and outside. It'd been the first time in a week I breathed in fresh air. It was raining, a light drizzle that'd felt like a gift from heaven - showering me with love.

*\*\*Sullivan District Hospital Neurology Ward, August 24,*

*2018\*\**

I'd never seen the monitoring room before. I thought it was new. But it had been there back in August 2015 during my three-week incarceration. It's a large room, the size of a whole ward, complete with a bathroom and shower. A window at the far end has a view of the North Shore mountains visible beyond the congested streets and tall buildings on the north side of the Seymour River. I placed my belongings in a new set of drawers and cupboards and changed into a clean hospital gown and robe. It was August 24th, one week from my status event and twenty-one seizures since.

I recognized her as she'd entered the room. Dr. Edwards's EEG technologist, Debra.

"Hi there. We need to get you set up. Would you follow me, please?"

In the room next to mine, she had me sit while she gathered her instruments and cables. Her technique wasn't any different from Foothills. The usual smelly airplane glue adhered the electrodes to my scalp—a woven mesh stretched over the top with more adhesive sprayed on with something akin to an airbrush. All wired up, she handed me a black pouch resembling a fanny pack. The wires that dangled off of my head fed into the side and connected to the Walkman type-box, and fastened to my waist. That was it: no jeopardy button to push, no screen to watch. They recorded everything in the tiny box strapped to my waist and sheets of paper and a pen to document my movements, such as going to the bathroom, eating, walking and standing. It was an archaic manual process compared to what I'd experienced at Foothills, but it had one advantage. I wasn't tethered to a computer; I could walk around the entire room, but I couldn't stand at the window. The only design flaw of the room had been where they'd mounted the camera. It's one hundred and eighty-degree views hadn't extended to the window. If I'd had a seizure while staring outside, the camera couldn't have recorded it. I knew the importance of staying within range and had deprived myself of the filtered daylight.

They had wired me up for two days before a neurologist saw me.

"Hello Linda, I know I'm no Dr. Edwards or Young, but I treat epilepsy." He settled himself on the chair across from me. "So, what we're going to do here is track you on the EEG for a few days. Let us know if you have questions." He stood and headed for the door.

*Well, uh, duh. Didn't he see all the wires coming from my head?* The ungracious thoughts ran through my mind, and it took a lot not to roll my eyes. My insides crumbled into a heap of despair as I watched him leave. *Is that it? Not asking how I was doing? Or discuss what has been going on?* I wished that Dr. Edwards was there, or I was in Foothills. It felt like the doctors and nurses were going through the motions of primary care. Crossing T's and dotting I's covering their asses, not sure what to do about me.

The seizures increased in number and length. Over the three days, I had eleven seizures, by my count, that lasted anywhere from thirty to forty-five minutes. My body was in the throes of an all-out war. Fatigue had set in, which made matters worse. Sleep deprivation is a trigger for me and I was fighting an endless battle. My faith in my caregivers faltered during one episode. I don't know how many nurses had answered my call bell, but when I heard the comment, "She's not shaking. I thought she'd be shaking. Is she having a seizure?" I panicked. I may not have heard correctly. Because how could a nurse work on a neurological ward and not know the different seizures? I felt helpless. There I was; stuck with the same doctors from 2015 and had felt like I'd fallen into a rabbit hole with no way out.—the dirt crumbling under my fingers not giving me the leverage I needed to climb up. 'My God. Oh Lord, please help me.'

**Discharged—Back to Community Hospital**

For forty-five minutes it went on. I was aware of my surroundings, but couldn't speak or control my body. Whether I passed out, or merely slipped away, it drew me into a void — the grasp on the here and now had disappeared, slid into a place of stillness, quiet peace, and nothingness. I told no one I wanted to go, to escape, to end my plight, and still my mind. I just wanted it to end.

While I lied in the hospital, the days combined and molded together and became one big smudge. When the nurse informed me of the transfer back, I froze. A cold sweat broke out, spread throughout my body and taken my blood away as it receded. Her words left me shaken and weak.

"What? Why are they transferring me back?" My stomach muscles clenched, and I felt my shoulders tense up. My heart raced and my breath came in quick short bursts, on the verge of hyperventilating.

"Didn't Dr. Dondel tell you? No, I guess he didn't." She rolled her eyes and muttered under her breath. "Ok, well, don't shoot the messenger, but the plan was for you to come for the EEG monitoring, then send you back. That's the only reason you're here."

My mouth dropped. I sat paralyzed shaking my head. I looked at her, the floor, the bed, up at the camera and back. Her words echoed throughout my head, just beyond my reach. It took two or three minutes before I finally grasped what her words meant. I wasn't admitted to Sullivan as a long-term patient. I'd been 'booked' into the seizure room for a test - nothing more. "No one told me that. When am I going?" The cold sweat heated and became a raging fire. 'I couldn't go back there. They didn't know what they're doing.' I was doomed and the panic inside me had taken over–my chest constricted, stomach muscles clenched tight, the tension radiated up to the shoulders, down my back through the flesh of my ass and down the legs. I thought I'd remain at Sullivan, that Dr. Edwards, my white knight, would've ridden in and made it go away. It had never occurred to me that my stay would only be temporary, and I'd be returned to the Community Hospital, which has no neurological ward nor a full-time neurologist. I felt like a hot potato that'd been tossed from doctor to doctor–a live grenade no one wanted to be holding when it went off.

"The transport vehicle is coming this evening sometime. It could be late, though. Pack your things up now, so you're ready when they get here." The nurse patted my leg, freshened my water, and handed me a package of cookies she'd grabbed from the kitchen. She then patted my arm, smiled and wished me luck.

The transfer occurred in the wee hours of the morning. Loaded up on a stretcher, my belongings back in bags, the ambulance drove through the night. By the time the paramedics unloaded me, it was 3 am Sunday, September 1st. I was well on my way to breaking my record of three weeks in the hospital — I was at two weeks and counting. They took me to a different wing of the hospital. I had a private room with its own toilet and shower. The window afforded a view of the city that had once been a small, quaint seaside town. Through the scratched and filthy window, I stared at the tall towers being constructed along Johnston Road. Cranes dotted the sky. Gone were most of the low-rise buildings that'd held the family businesses from my youth. The gas station on the corner and the butcher shop, a few doors down, had become a massive hole bordered by concrete walls, rebars, and a cement floor. It didn't help to improve my mood.

I occupied my time, sitting up in bed, updating my tracking calendars and writing in my notebook. By then, I'd had thirty-eight seizures since August 17th. It'd averaged out to three per day.

# Chapter Sixteen

## **Sea of Beds**

*Living amongst a sea of beds full of poor souls, Lost—lonely, trapped in their own worlds. Places we will never see, can't be nor follow, their destinations are exclusive - Private, Availability just for one. Those of us on the fringe, Wonder—Worry—Conjecture. Must use our imaginations to peer through their eyes, See what's on the other side. Some are quiet—Serene—Lost in a dream, Others—Angry—Frustrated - Violent. Crying out loud—Screaming and afraid. Terrifying nightmares torture their beings. There I lay, In my room with a view Exhausted—Lonely—Frightened. Caught in my own torment of pain, Confusion—Frustration—Loneliness; Despair. Living between Past and Present, no Future yet to see. Our paths quite similar, Although They're further along. Kindred Spirits amongst a sea of beds, trapped in our minds with nowhere to go.\**

They placed me in an area reserved for the elderly — those with mobility difficulties and dementia. My neighbour

Viola was a sweet dear lady lost from reality. I will never forget the day she wheeled herself into my room, begging me to help her.

"Can you get this off me? I can't seem to remove it. I need to get it off so I can get in the car. I can't get in the car with it on." Her hands clamped around the buckle of a seat belt, its purpose to keep her strapped in the wheelchair. It had no push-button release like a standard belt. It required a slim, sharp object inserted into a small hole to undo the clasp. I felt sorry for her situation and how she was losing her mind. In a soft voice, I suggested,

"Why don't you go find the nurse? She can help you get out. You need a special tool to remove your seatbelt. Sorry, Viola, I can't help you." I pointed to the hole in the middle of the buckle, then patted her hand.

"I need to get this off. Peter can't get me in the car with it on." She sounded so sad as she pushed herself out of my room. She used her feet to push herself along backwards. I knew the chances of them undoing her belt were slim. Her bed alarm went off day and night as she would forget where she was and fall out or wander. Viola, I could handle. It was the screams and moans from the other side of the ward that got to me. Poor souls in excruciating pain, minds tormented by hallucinations as their dementia worsened.

Caught in my own battles of mind over body, I continued to seize. Surrounded by caregivers oozing with empathy and sympathetic to my needs—but the lack of experience still existed. Nurses witnessing events would come in and say, "Oh, you're having one of them silent seizures." No one seemed to know what to do with me. I felt lost in a sea of beds. My emotions ran at turbo speed, and I resumed journaling and poetry. I hadn't written poems in years, not since my teens. I had always been better at expressing myself through writing. Jotting down my thoughts was excellent therapy for my heart and soul. It was during this time I wrote Sea of Beds. I believed I would never get out of there, stuck just as my roomies were. But that didn't happen. My next seizure put the wheel in motion that released me.

I heard movement out in the ward. Nurses were talking, giving instructions and sounding exasperated with their charges. I found out later they were shifting beds around. Why? I don't know. During their spring clean, a seizure struck. I pressed the call button when it didn't stop. My body seemed frozen, and it was a struggle to reach down and grab the call bell that had slipped off the bed to the floor. I heard it ringing above the commotion. Then it stopped. Expecting a nurse to arrive, I waited. No one showed up. I pressed the button again.

Heard it ring, then stopped. Was it possible they couldn't hear it ringing? I picked up my water jug and hurled it towards the open doorway. It hit the wall and bounced back inside, dumping its contents. The seizure wasn't stopping, and I panicked. I pushed the button once more. I could hear it above the racket, but the nurses couldn't? It stopped again. The clock on the wall ticked away; the seizure had been going almost thirty minutes, and I was losing strength. I remember yelling, but my voice was caught in my throat, came out more as a croak and wasn't much above a whisper. Then Dr. Breen walked in. He stepped over the jug and pool of water at the door, his eyes on me as he came to the bedside. He took my wrist, had placed his fingers on the pulse and watched my face as he counted the beats. I'd been seizing for over thirty minutes, had tried calling the nurses three times, but no one had come. I croaked out. Tears flowed, and my body had shaken with the strain of my situation. He spun on his heels, was out the door and strode down the hallway to the nurses' station, calling for Ativan. *Stat.* A nurse scurried into my room, shoved a pill under my tongue and darted out. As the seizure subsided, I curled into a ball. My breath had slowed, and I felt the tension recede, but my emotional state had remained in overdrive. Dr. Breen found me gasping for air as the sobs wracked my body.

"What's wrong, Ms. McClure? You're ok now." He watched me intently, glancing at the monitors and back to my face.

"I-I-I thought I-I-I w-w-a-s going to die." My head lifted an inch or two from its nest amongst the pillows. He patted my shoulder, uttered a few soothing words to calm me. I must have fallen asleep afterwards. When I woke up, he had gone.

Dr. Breen returned later that day and informed me he hadn't heard from Dr. Edwards. That he was waiting for him to read the EEG. And that the only neurologist to have visited me hadn't wanted to get involved. 'Too many cooks in the kitchen," he said. The current neurologist on call had suggested to him that that was most likely my new norm. *What*? Was this neurologist making a prognosis without having seen me? *Where the fuck was Dr. Edwards*?

"Have you spoken to Dr. Young?" I asked Dr. Breen.

"Who's that?" his eyebrow cocked as he thumbed through my chart.

"He's my neurologist in Calgary. His number should be in there. Dr. Chung spoke with him when I was first here." *How did he miss that? Did he not read the notes?*

274

"What's his number? I'll keep trying Dr. Edwards, but will call this Dr. Young in the meantime." Fumbling around for my phone, I recited the number for him to call.

"Leave a message, and he'll call you back." I sank back on the bed and closed my eyes. Dr. Young would set them all straight. He was my lifeline, my only hope to get out of this mess. It was amazing how the thought of Dr. Young and Foothills had calmed me. Just envisioning the SMU, the nurses, technologists, and team of doctors and surgeons, had been enough to slow my ragged breathing, reduced my booming heart to a dull thump, and blanketed me with a soft glow of warmth and security. When Dr. Breen had left, I'd sent one last email to Dr. Edwards for help.

*From: Linda McClure*

*Sent: September 6, 2018 4:51 PM*

*To: Dr. Edwards*

*Subject: McClure Linda SEIZURE & HOSPITAL STATUS please help*

*Dear Dr. Edwards*

*I'm writing to you in desperation, frustration and complete exhaustion.*

*Since my status event on August 17th that dumped me into the Community Hospital, my situation went from bad to worse. What started as a onetime event progressed to daily seizures with some lasting upwards of 30 minutes.*

*August 19 - 2?*

*August 20 - 3*

*August 21 - 2*

*August 22 - 3*

*August 23–3*

*August 24 - 4*

*August 25 - 3*

*August 26 - 2*

*Plus the ones captured on the EEG. The total for the month of August is about 40 seizures!!*

*September has continued with an average of 2 per day.*

*Even with Dr. Young's help, all eyes are turning to you, to:*

*1. Interpret the EEG*

*2. Provide your input as my neurologist to work together to determine my plan of care when, what, and how to proceed upon my discharge.*

*During my 3 weeks of hospitalization, I've seen a neurologist once for a brief visit prior to the EEG. Nothing's been communicated with as to any plans for my care or release beyond the tapering of the Lacosamide as per Dr. Young's orders.*

*No one wants to take responsibility or be accountable for making these decisions in my case.*

*I'm an anomaly to them. Most nurses at both Community & Sullivan District have never seen my type of seizures before. I'm a freak show that everybody wants to peek at, but not get too close to.*

*Please, please take a moment to change hats and help me out. If you could return Dr. B's message (he's the hospitalist this week) that would be a great help.*

*Thanking you in advance.*

*Sincerely,*

*Linda McClure*

I must have drifted off when my phone rang. Foothills splashed across the screen. *Thank God.* "Hello?"

"Hi, Ms. McClure. Dr. Young here. How are you feeling?" Not waiting for an answer, he continued. "Listen, Dr. Breen and I agree that the best thing to do is bring you here to Calgary. We've got a bed in the unit for you." He paused as if consulting his notes. "We can do this one of two ways. By a hospital transfer or you can get here on your own. Whichever is easier. Which do you want to do?" My reply had been immediate.

"It would be easiest to do a hospital transfer; otherwise, I'd have to find someone to go with me. Dr. Young? I'm sorry to have involved you, but I had no one else. Dr. Edwards is *away*." My heart overflowed with gratitude. It filled to where tears formed and huge droplets fell onto my notebook, hands and blanket.

"It's ok, Ms. McClure. Only it's difficult for me to consult from here. Bringing you into the seizure unit is the best option to help you out. So, you want to come via hospital transfer then? You won't be under my name, but we'll sort that out on our end. We'll see you soon." The pressure on my shoulders and the binding around my chest lifted, and my heart soared. I was going to get the help I needed. I was going back to the SMU, my second home.

The first call I made was the Epilepsy Clinic. The next had been to my sister. She knew how to arrange the transfer; as a nurse practitioner, she'd done them before and in her no nonsense take charge and get er done style, she took care of the finer details. There had been a few hiccups, however, and more phone calls made back and forth to Calgary, but it'd sorted out and I left via the medevac on the following Sunday.

*September 9, 2018 Foothills Seizure Monitoring Unit*

*(SMU)—Fancy seeing you again*

I knew what to bring, but it was hard trying to convey my instructions on where to find everything to Devon, who volunteered to help. A carry-on bag and shopping bags held a change of clothes, pyjamas, toiletries, puzzle books, and some healthy snacks. Mom had taken what clothing I'd been toting around and washed them, returning them neatly folded. Packed up and ready to leave the nightmare behind me, the paramedics took me down to the waiting ambulance. The fresh air, even with the smell of exhaust, had been divine after three weeks of breathing recycled hospital air.

We drove to the Vancouver International airport, arriving at the south terminal where smaller planes and cargo jets are, and pulled up next to the medevac on the tarmac. I assumed I would be in a seat, but that wasn't the case. They deposited me inside, stretcher and all. There were no seats on one side of the carrier to accommodate my prone position, and the stretcher buckled in to keep it from shifting during the flight. My attendants took their seats across from me, one in front of the other. The cramped space of the aircraft couldn't accommodate rows like you'd find in a commercial or private plane. The two seats and the pilots were the only ones leaving room for my stretcher, bags, and the EMT equipment. Each passenger had their own window, but not the luxury of much leg room. They had given me a dose of Ativan before we'd left the hospital to thwart off the possibility of any seizures during the flight. The paramedics remained with me until we landed and had passed me off to their Calgary counterparts, then returned to BC. How it all worked was fascinating—my removal from the plane to the waiting ambulance–the transfer of information and the ride to Foothills.

It was my fourth visit to the unit, and I'd become well known to the staff. If I'd had a dollar for how often I'd heard, "Oh, you're back?" I could've bought coffee for the entire eleventh floor. They gave me the same cell I'd had last November for the intracranial monitoring. It didn't take long to unpack the few belongings I'd brought. I arranged the carry-on full of clothes, the snacks, and toiletries along the window ledge, positioning them within easy reach from the bed. The same pyjamas I'd worn the previous year hung a little looser on me. Before I settled in for a much-needed nap, Olivia attached the electrodes. Down the familiar hallway lined with discarded equipment and broken furniture to the same room as on my previous visits. Airplane glue, wires, and lots of cables were arranged on the counter. I laid on the table with a rolled-up towel under my neck for support and chatted away as Olivia worked. She asked what had brought me back into the unit and

I told her what had happened, that I'd been in hospital since the 17th of August and how I'd gotten to Foothills. She couldn't believe what had happened and how I'd ended up there. My braid of wires glued to my head and hanging down between my breasts was comforting. The pouch that sat on my shoulder and slung across by breast holding the wires had soothed me. Back to my room, Olivia hooked me up to the computer mounted on the wall.

"Ok, Linda, you know the drill. Open your eyes. Now close them. Good. Once more. Open. Close. Okay, press the button, please." She scooted to the open door and called out, "Test." Satisfied all was in order, she'd headed off for her break. "See ya later."

Gluing the electrodes to my skull I referred to as becoming the Bride of Frankenstein. Humour had always been my way to armour myself against the harsh realities of life and then had been no exception. Scared, terrified, and emotionally scarred by these events - bounced from hospital to hospital, visited by doctor A, B, C, D, E and so on. It felt like I was on a conveyor belt being pieced together, only to find the parts were faulty and I'd malfunctioned. I would later describe those weeks as traumatizing. Which they had been. To have not felt comfortable in my hometown had been unthinkable. That they hadn't known what to do with me and, worse, couldn't have done anything to help me, had appalled and angered me. My condition baffled them, and there hadn't been the resources, knowledge, or expertise to provide the level of care I'd needed. I hadn't felt safe, and in my mind, had been lucky to have survived. Foothills and Calgary are my saving grace. The people, the knowledge and expertise have granted me the serenity I've needed to stay sane. It's sad I've felt more at home and safer there than anywhere else.


But my return to the fold hadn't calmed the storm that railed within. Two seizures hit that first day and with no reduction in meds. After three weeks of hospitalization, it was essential to figure out the source; why they'd ramped up. The team reduced my medications the next day. It took four days before a clear reading on the EEG would surface. It was small but was a start. On the fifth day, during my PET scan (positron emission tomography scan) I had one of my waves. They had injected me with a radioactive drug known as radiotracers to visualize and measure the physiological activities within my body. The procedure produces three-dimensional images of the blood flow, chemical reactions and muscular activity as they occur in the brain. It measured the metabolism of my glucose and oxygen and would reveal the active areas with increased blood flow and higher consumption of oxygen. These measurements would help to locate the site from which my seizures originated from. I was inside the scanner when it occurred. Eyes closed; I breathed through it as the tide washed over me. It was difficult not to move as it hit, but somehow I managed it.

Over the next four days, I endured nine seizures, countless waves, ghostly images, nausea, and anxiety. My vision was distorted, and I'd read the digital clock above my door as 6:30 vs 9:30. I heard my phone ring when it hadn't and even held conversations with people that weren't there–asked my imaginary friend if he knew the title of the song that'd been playing and whether they liked it. I would feel lightheaded–my head all floaty like a lonely helium balloon pushed back and forth and up and down by the slightest movement. My arms and legs would become tingly as if they'd just awoken–encased in pins and needles making them numb. My speech slowed and became slurred–headaches were constant. The days ticked over from one to the next with no respite from these sensations wrapped around me. They were relentless.

On September 17th, I had a SPECT scan. And just as they had done on my first visit to the SMU, they injected me with radioactive dye and inserted me into the scanner. I'd had my typical waves plus two seizures that day, which had made it easy to perform the test.

*September 18 to 19, 2018 Status Epilepticus #1*

I would spend my days reading, writing, Netflix bingeing, and watching the helicopter take off and land—bringing trauma cases from outlying areas. Nineteen seizures during that first week hadn't produced enough sufficient data. Ten days in, we then tried sleep-deprivation. Lack of sleep is one of my triggers that stirs the pot and causes a tornado effect within the confines of my skull. That time was no different, except I went into status.

[Status Epilepticus: A prolonged seizure lasting more than thirty minutes; or a cluster of seizures occurring one after the other without recovering in between. Considered a medical emergency. Can cause severe brain damage or death.]

For three hours, I seized. Audrey, my nurse, was beside herself. Her calls to Dr. Norris had kept him awake throughout the night, as his concern for my well-being mounted. Dr. Norris is the senior member of the team, having been at Foothills since the 80s. Shorter and older than his male counterparts, he brought years of experience with epilepsy, sleep disorders, and multiple sclerosis. He felt like an uncle to me. I derived much comfort from his calm demeanour and realistic advice. I grew quite fond of him and enjoyed his visits.

I was on my side, trying to go to sleep when it occurred. My mouth overflowed with saliva and soaked into the pillow, followed by chewing motions. I pressed the button, setting off the alarm which summoned Audrey. Everything went dark after she arrived. She said she performed the usual tests: "What's your name? Where are you? Who am I?" Asked me to point at things. Remember this word, a colour, squeeze my fingers, push your feet down onto my hands, then push up. I had entered my blank space, my world where no one could follow, and I'd taken my time coming back.

The next day I wouldn't move off the bed other than to pee, so exhausted was my body; it took an effort to eat. The simple act of moving fork and spoon from plate or bowl to mouth and back was like asking a Boston Marathoner to turn around and go again.

Inflammation of the brain and autoimmune diseases can cause seizures but is treated far easier than epilepsy. I had a lumbar puncture to extract spinal fluid to send for testing the day after my status event. I'd always been a challenge for the doctors to insert the needle into position to extract the spinal fluid. An ultrasound machine was used to guide the doctor as the needle punctured through skin and muscle and into the cord, withdrawing the fluid. This procedure can cause back pain and migraine type headaches. My back wasn't bad, but my head was a different matter. With the constant changes in barometric pressure, I suffered more from the weather than the lumbar. Tylenol and laying down with eyes closed was my only recourse; that, and time. They'd sent the fluid plus blood samples down to the Mayo Clinic. If there was anything untoward going on, they would have found it. But just as with the previous ones, the test came back clear.

I'd now been in hospital for over a month — twenty-two days back at home and fifteen days in the SMU–a record for me.

Dr. Norris's rotation ended, and Dr. Isaacs's began. I'd met her back in November when I had the intra cranial monitoring. She appeared younger than the other team members. Slight of frame, smooth complexion and beautiful wrinkle-free eyes, she could've passed as a med student. Before Dr. Norris had departed, he asked me if I'd do him a favour. Dr. O'Connor had wanted to bring his students in and perform a hands-on exam. Besides being involved in the epilepsy program, he's also an Associate Professor at the University of Calgary. All I had to do was sit there and undergo simple tests such as squeeze their hands and push up and down against their palms with my feet and follow a pen with my eyes. Nothing that I hadn't been through before. Thankful to them all for everything they'd done for me, I had agreed. Besides, I had plenty of time on my hands.


Dr. O'Connor arrived with half a dozen students. It felt like I was a lab specimen as they surrounded my bed and stared down at me. Their job was to interview me; get my medical history and perform the physical exam. Soon word had spread that there was a patient in the SMU who will talk about her epilepsy. The next to visit was a neurologist, who wasn't part of the team associated with the unit. Again, needing a change of pace from TV, puzzle books, FB, and poetry, I agreed to be his human specimen. I regaled them with my story, including the good and the not so good. Their visit was too short and alone once again. I returned to Netflix. I'd read a book earlier in the year called Brain on Fire, My Month of Madness by Susannah Cahalan, and had discovered the movie on Netflix. Her story about NMDA receptor encephalitis, a rare autoimmune disease, was a gripping tale of her trials of misdiagnosis and subsequent recovery. While our conditions had differed, her experiences hit close to home. I felt her terror; her frightened feelings, depression, and anxiety. I related to the medical system working against her. The movie brought home all the emotion I carried. Feelings of sadness weighing me down, not knowing if I had the strength to make it. I enjoyed the movie but hadn't struck a chord with me as the book had. A few of the nurses told me they had read the book to gain insight into the patient's perspective. They were trained to watch, wait, and react. Patients would answer their inquiries about symptoms and what they felt. The nurses' focus is on how to treat the physical, leaving the mental state for the counsellors and psychologists. I would soon discover that Foothills provided a buffet of options that were limited at home and still are at the time of writing my story.

They forewarned me upon my admittance that I'd have to move rooms to make way for a surgical patient. I'd entered my second week at Foothills when I moved to bed A. My new cell was smaller than the one I'd just vacated but was closer to the nurses' station, mini fridge, coffeemaker, and microwave, which had suited me just fine. I was now within reach of my two favourite beverages, coffee and water, and could serve myself.

I continued being the test subject for the professors, with Dr. Young being the last to bring his gaggle of would-be doctors. I saw a different side of him - always professional with his patients. He was more relaxed. He had a good rapport with his students, and I could tell they looked up to him. To lecture his students from a podium hadn't the same complications that came within a hospital setting. After the students had filed out, he hung back to see how I'd been managing.

"So, how are you holding up, Linda?"

"Okay, all things considered." I waved my arms around the room Vanna-style and grinned.

"Listen, we're not getting the readings we'd hoped to get. I wanted to see what your thoughts were on proceeding to depth probes. As you know from before, we need to get deeper into your brain to locate the seizure focus. Are you open to that?"

"Yes."

"Good. Good." He patted my leg and turned to leave.

"Dr. Young?"

He turned back and stood at the end of my bed.

"Thank you for taking the time to look after me. Everyone here has been incredible. I don't know what I'd have done without you. I'm very fortunate to have you as my doctor. You're an important man, and I'm thankful for the time you've given me. You and Dr. Edwards have been my lifelines throughout this." I choked up as I spoke–the emotions I'd kept hidden exposed. He smiled and nodded.

"I'm only important to my family. We'll let you know when the surgery will be. Take care, Linda." As I watched him leave, I relaxed against the pillows, pulled my knees up and wrapped my arms around them - hugging myself to release the tension of my lower back, letting out a long sigh of contentment.

[I'd always been a believer that *Everything happens for a reason, and there's a reason things happen, but it hadn't hit home until then. I was here for treatment, yes, but I was giving back as well. It had felt good to play the guinea pig and, hopefully, provide these upcoming doctors with some additional knowledge about seizures and epilepsy.*]

It may have been the same day or the next when the neurosurgeon, Dr. Ingals, introduced himself. With his briefcase in hand and a team member fast on his heels, he knocked and entered my room.

"Hi. I'm Dr. Ingals. I'm to perform the surgery to insert your depth probes and have some time available on October 2nd if you're up to it. You should know that my procedure is different from Dr. Taylor's. I use a robotic arm and we bolt the electrodes in place versus stitched. I use a general anesthetic so you'd be out during the operation. Do you have any questions?" His dark hair and healthy tan had made him appear younger. He exuded confidence and charm, and I had no qualms with him performing the procedure.

"No, no questions. Where do I sign?" His eyes widened and brows lifted as he turned to the fellow beside him, reaching for the forms held in his hand. I don't think he'd had a patient sign so quickly. I merely glanced over the paper, not paying attention to the fine print. I'd been through it before and was comfortable signing it. I scribbled my signature and held up the paper. He took the proffered form, shook my hand, and bid me farewell.

"That was easy." He commented to his cohort.

I felt strange after they left. Dr. Taylor had been there from the beginning. He had performed both resections and the intracranial so far and felt as if I'd cheated on him.

My seizure activity had been dropping off by then, and I felt almost normal. Dr. O'Connor, who was on shift that week, had come by and informed me they would remove my leash. I'd have the weekend untethered.

"Enjoy your freedom, Linda. Come Monday night, I'm taking away your get out of jail free card."

"Oh, so I can wander anywhere?" I chuckled.

"Only on this floor." His eyes crinkled when he smiled, then had disappeared as the humour had left his voice. "I'm serious, Linda. You need to stay on this floor. Okay? Enjoy your weekend off." I realized after he'd left that without the electrodes I got to shower!

I'd now spent forty days in the hospital and had loved that I could roam around beyond the confines of the SMU. I walked as much as I could. Out the door of the unit, I'd pass the nurses' station, swung right, strolled down the corridor past the kitchen and shower room down to the end. Another right took me past beds separated by drapes and turned up the next corridor back to the unit. Around and around I wandered side-stepping mobile computer stations, blood pressure machines, laundry and meal carts, and the constant stream of doctors and nurses. When I'd tired of that, I would sit on the stationary bike parked in front of the nurse's station, pedalling and chatting to whoever had felt like talking. My goal was twenty minutes per session. I didn't want to sweat too much since my supply of clean clothes had depleted. But I needed to move. I could've been there another two weeks before they had gathered enough information to sort me out. And if another resection had been necessary, I could be there even longer. It had reached a point where no amount of deodorant could hide the smell of sweat on my pyjamas. Without my family close by, I took matters into my own hands. Outside my room was a large sink with a soap dispenser attached to the wall. Who needed a machine when I could hand wash? I spent a good part of that weekend washing tops, pants, underwear, and socks. My room had looked like a back alley strung with drying laundry. Shirts hung on hooks in the cupboard and on the wall by the door; underwear and socks had decorated the shelves. As each piece dried, another took its place.

"I've always said we should have one of those all-in-one washer-dryers in here. For cases like yours." Carrie said after watching the toils of my labour.

"Well, it's kept me busy." I headed to the fridge to get more water and found only one left. "Do you want me to go get more water? There's one left, and I seem to drink most of it." I grabbed the tray I'd seen the nurses use and side shuffled towards the open doorway.

"Sure, if you like, that would be great."

"Where do I go?" My face broke into a grin, and I felt light and carefree at the prospect of escape.

"Take a right at the nurses' station. Another right, and not far down on your right, is a kitchen area. Cups, lids, and straws are on the counter. If there isn't enough, then check the cupboards. You know you don't have to do it." Relaxing back in her chair, her hand on the phone, she waited to see if I'd change my mind.

"Sure, I do. I need to earn my keep. Besides, it'll allow me to stretch my legs. Back in a minute." I scurried towards the opening when her voice halted my exit. Drat. Chest deflated and shoulders slumped, I faced my jailor.

"Oh, and tell them I let you go." I gave her a thumbs up and headed out of the unit, feeling important. It made sense for me to help. The nurses couldn't leave without calling someone to come in and cover. With replenishing water, they relied upon the other nurses to bring it when they had a moment. By my helping, it didn't disrupt the routine or take a nurse away from other patients in need. I was alongside the station when a voice stopped me.

"Are you allowed out?" I turned toward the desk, ready for a fight. "Yes, I'm getting water for the unit." I held up the tray to prove my point, and that I wasn't lying.

"Uh-huh. So you say." Oscar looked at me as if I was a child trying to put one over on a parent. "Why aren't you hooked up?" He motioned with his head to my scalp, devoid of wires; Eyebrow raised, he became suspicious and questioning my motives.

"I'm getting depth probes inserted on Tuesday. Dr. O'Connor has given me the weekend off before I'm tethered to my bed again." He thought a moment, considering my answer. Satisfied, he came round to my side and led the way to the kitchen.

"If you need more cups, you can find them here." Opening a cupboard and drawers, he gave me a quick tour.

"Thanks." My tray ladened with Styrofoam cups full of water and ice and, careful not to spill, I made my way back.

"What's this?" I glanced up, standing still so I wouldn't spill.

"I'm paying for my keep." Dr. O'Connor looked at Carrie and then at the tray. Turning aside, shaking his head and hiding a smile, I made my way to the fridge. I found room for all but one, which I took to my room. And so I went back and forth, keeping our fridge stocked and handing out water to my roommates. I felt the best that I had since this all started. My spirits lifted somewhat from the depths to which they had fallen. Monday came too suddenly, but I got to shower before heading into the OR. I've never appreciated the luxury of soap and water and clean hair until I came to the unit. The patient in the next room had packed up and left, so once again, I shifted rooms. I will now have been in every bed in the unit. I joked about how it had to be a record or I belonged to an elite club.

That Dr. Edwards wasn't in the picture at a time I could have used him was disconcerting. Our patient-doctor relationship had grown. I could communicate with him via email between office visits. To me, he had become my confidant, a friend. His silence worried me to the point I had him lying in a hospital ill

with some grave disease, dying.

# Chapter Seventeen


## **The Nuts and Bolts and Surgery**

*October 2, 2018,* and I was back in the OR once again. It was getting monotonous. Dr. Ingals reminded me that his procedure differed from that of Dr. Taylor's. He uses a robotic arm to insert the probes and bolts versus stitches. He referred to her as Rosa. I'm sure it meant something, but I couldn't get rid of the image of Rosie, the robotic housemaid from the Jetsons. This time I was in a different holding bay, jam-packed with row upon row of beds. Getting a nurses' attention was a challenge, as they'd raced around from bed to bed. I had to go pee and didn't know where to go. With only minutes before they'd take me in, I flagged a nurse and she escorted me to the washroom. She waited outside the door and as I emerged; she whisked me away into the OR. That time, I didn't have to listen to the whirr of a drill or feel its pressure as it broke through bone and brain matter. As with my first two surgeries, they positioned my head, supported my neck with foam and a towel, then clamped it in to keep it from moving. Straps like seat belts attached to the bottom of the table wrapped up and over my torso and buckled. I looked like a mummy from the neck down my left arm and head left exposed. The anesthesiologist inserted the IV, covered my mouth and nose with a mask.

"Okay, Linda. I want you to breathe in deeply. I'm going to administer a mild sedative in to the IV. You may feel a cold, burning sensation. That's it, keep breathing...." And... gone.

I came to in recovery, with a headache no worse than I'd experienced before. I'd become used to the post surgery effects. Thirteen probes covered the right side of my head from front to back. My shaved head was like a desecrated forest of stumps dotting the landscape. Back in my room, Olivia hooked me up to my old buddy, Wall-E. She wrapped my head in material similar to that of a tensor bandage, but instead of the standard beige, it was bright pink. I looked like I had one of those pink marshmallow candies plopped onto my head. Brightly coloured and cheery, it made everyone smile, except me. I hated pink, despised it. It figured Olivia had chosen it for me.

Without missing a beat, the next round of students came to watch the monkey in the cage. They belonged to Dr. Irwin, a semi-retired member of the epilepsy team and a professor at the University of Calgary. In my previous visits, I'd never met him, which had been ironic, as he was the doctor I was to have had my initial consultation with back in 2016. But that never occurred; I'd bypassed that step and came straight in for monitoring. Dr. Irwin and his students hadn't waited long before my show begun. A facial tick and slurred speech, and body twitches - a repeat of my previous performances for their private viewing. The ghost images would come and go but had never left. The same day Dr. Irwin had come by, I'd seen the outline of my nurse as she'd left her image burned into my cornea - a ghostly image remained even after I closed my eyes. It took me back to August 2015 when the shape of a nurse stood in my doorway when, in fact, he'd been across the hall. It'd been just as unsettling then, as it had the first time. Seizure activity? Not sure, but I thought I lost my mind when two of Dr. Ingals' surgical team came to discuss my ghost images, vision deficiency, and placement of my electrodes. The team ordered a CT scan, and another round in the donut hole had confirmed no further holes had been necessary since the EEG wasn't picking up the ghost images and, as I would later discover, was because I was getting old. As my brain got older, it couldn't relay the changes in light at the same speed, which caused a blurred after image like that of a double exposed picture.

We had hoped to perform surgery on the eleventh once they captured another two solid seizure readings. Alas, no one had sent the memo to my brain, and it failed to comply. Not that there had been no seizures—they just hadn't registered on the EEG. I had then been in the hospital for fifty-eight consecutive days - thirty-five of them spent in Foothills alone. After living off hospital food, with little to no exercise other than to the washroom and the odd spin on the exercise bike, my daily constitution suffered. I experienced stomach issues– nausea, bloating, and pains. I battled diarrhea, then constipation, and when I thought things were back in working order, the diarrhea would start up again. My focus had shifted from head to torso—distracting my brain from the task at hand. I tried to stress myself out. I even called the friend who'd had triggered a seizure the last time we'd talked on the phone. But it hadn't worked. When we eliminated my dose of Dilantin, I had thought for sure we would've seen some action. But nothing happened. They had given me the weekend up to the following Tuesday to produce something. If successful, they would discuss my case at the committee meeting with surgery as early as that Thursday. I was desperate to give them what they wanted. I wanted to end the torture and make it go away. The only thing we hadn't tried was sleep deprivation. It had worked before, so why wouldn't it then? I volunteered, hoping it would work.

The night of my self-induced sleep deprivation, I had a fully charged tablet, downloaded several Netflix shows, a deck of cards, and pen and paper. At dinner, I chugged back steaming hot coffee, refilling my oversized Styrofoam cup from the carafe outside my room multiple times. Determined to squeeze out a whopper, I did whatever I could've to trip that wire, pull the brass ring, and detonate the charge. Whatever it had been. The caffeine. The hours spent forcing my eyes to keep open had worked. My thumb and index finger began rubbing together. A repetitive motion over which I had no control. What happened after that? I do not know. Small clips like movie scenes surface once in a while, but nothing clear. That night is blurry, like a smudged fingerprint left on the lens of a pair of glasses. Brief moments of clarity bring forth snippets of a memory. The recollection of a head twitching. Not in sync with the thumb and finger, moving at its own speed, jerky and slow. I awoke with a sore neck. The muscles twinged and popped just like kernels in hot oil. No amount of ice or heat eased it. Rest and time was the only option.

The good news: The EEG had captured what they wanted. They had all they needed to present to the committee on Thursday. The bad news: I'd gone into status. Poor Audrey was beside herself as she'd tried to bring me out of it. When told my seizure had run for almost six hours, I hadn't believed them. But it'd made sense. I felt like a zombie with a massive headache–dysfunctional. Depending on how you looked at it, Audrey was my good luck charm or a jinx. My status events only occurred on her watch. She'd been my trigger, that, or my brain had it in for her. Whatever the reason, I produced the required results to move forward with surgery.

The SPECT scan results showed the Insula was still creating issues and had lit up the screen. Same as it had back in June and November 2017. The committee was reluctant to remove it. The Insula has an intricate network of blood vessels surrounding it, and the probability of a stroke was real should one of them get nicked. And its removal could affect my left arm and leg. It would affect typing, day-to-day capabilities such as dressing could diminish, and, as Dr. Ingals had mentioned, 'I wouldn't be able to learn guitar.' The committee had determined the Insula would remain intact. The seizure had already created issues with my left hand and neck muscles, and I was still recovering from the aftereffects of the seizure itself. Knowing they wouldn't touch the insula had provided some comfort. Being told my seizure focus had spread was alarming. The surgical site would expand beyond the first and second operations, getting as close to the insula as possible.

**October 18, 2018—Third surgery–Foothills Medical Centre**

On a cold, narrow table, surrounded by nurses and the anaesthetist, they strapped me in and hooked me up to a myriad of machines and tubes. My head was placed in a cradle and situated for easy access, and locked in place, not allowing for the slightest of movements.

"Is there something massaging my left hand?" It lay upon an armrest. My fingers stroked in a soothing gesture. Or so I thought.

"No. What do you mean?" the Anesthetist asked.

"It feels like something is rubbing my fingers. I thought it was a special armrest or something."

"Nothing's touching your hand."

"Could it be a nerve thing? Like where they put the IV in?" Nothing was moving except what my mind had led me to believe. I've always been a problematic IV start; had they punctured a nerve when inserting the needle? They moved the

IV and carried on with their preparations. I'll never know if that had been the issue; I was out soon after.

Next thing I knew, I was in recovery. How long it'd taken, I've no clue. Dr. Ingals removed the electrodes as he'd cracked open my skull to take another chunk out. At least that's what I remember. The first time they'd removed the probes in the unit; cutting the stitches and pulling out the wires.

I've had many surgeries during my fifty-three years with no adverse side effects from the anaesthesia. That time was the exception. After settling in my room, I began throwing up with each contraction of my stomach, causing pain. Throughout the night, I retched. The pressure that built, rising from my gut, up the throat and out, had added to my discomfort. Once it'd subsided, I could only keep sips of water down. But even with that, I encountered difficulties. My thumb on my left hand couldn't grip the Styrofoam cup. It was as if it was dead. My motor skills had reverted to when I was a baby, learning to grasp and hold on to small objects. Grabbing a fork to cut up food was an exercise in futility and frustration. *Had I stroked during the surgery?* No. No, my left leg and arm were alright. Only my hand seemed to be an issue. And my mouth. The left corner drooped, and if I hadn't paid attention and focused on eating or drinking, the liquid and food would fall out. I dubbed it my dribble mouth. I was using towels as bibs to begin with, was careful while I ate and drank, trying hard not to mess up the sheets and blanket. As with the second surgery, the pain had been tolerable. The Tylenol had kept it from exploding out of control.

Dr. Ingals visited me two or three times before he discharged me six days post-op. He even came by on the Sunday to check up on me. I saw more of him post-surgery than any other surgeon who'd cut into my defenceless body. I could see why he worked at the Children's Hospital. It'd take a special individual to work with sick young children - patients who didn't understand what's going on and some too ill to have cared.

Each day that passed, my strength returned. When I could walk the corridors without using the walls and discarded equipment to steady myself, I knew it was time to think of going home. No seizures post surgery. The biggest concern I had was my hand. Only slightly improved, I still found it difficult to eat, hold a washcloth or towel, pickup and use a fork, or pulling the blankets around me at night. I had to focus on chewing and drinking, keeping the food and liquids from dribbling out the side of my mouth—landing on the tray or in my lap. Both the physical and occupational therapists examined me and determined I was fit to leave. It was time. Sixty-seven days. Forty-five of them in Foothills. As much as I wanted to go home, leaving my little cocoon was difficult, but I had to get home to my own space, my son Devon, our cat, Coco. It'd been hard on Dev to hold down the fort while I was hundreds of miles away and forced to manage the day-to-day responsibilities. Juggling home, work, a cat was a lot for a young man of 24 who'd never lived on his own.


*[The doctors, surgeons, and nurses at Foothills take their roles seriously. Their commitment, empathy, and understanding they'd extended to me, far exceeded the level of care I'd had at home, except for a few. They've seen me at my worst and most vulnerable, and I've never felt safer than I have at Foothills. It's my second home, and they're my extended family. It's because of that deep connection to the seizure unit and the staff that made it difficult to leave.]*

# Chapter Eighteen

## **November 2018—Back Home**

[My time spent at Foothills is a collection of short, quick images—jumbled up with memories of previous visits. Those trips to the seizure unit and the events during my 67-day stay are fragmented. In my mind's eye, they all appear in bursts like an old movie shown on a reel to reel. Picture–blank–image–image–snow–repeat - and fade to black. If it weren't for my calendars, my half-dozen notebooks and poetry, the chain of events would have gaps the size of the Pacific Ocean. No one else knows the full story, not family or friends. My doctors hold pieces of the puzzle, some more than others, and can recreate my journey to some extent. But I keep those last few pieces that bring the picture to life, and I alone can appreciate the story it conveys.]

***December 2018—Christmas**

That year we had a small gathering. Just five of us sat around Mom's dining room table. Margaret and Barry had cooked the bird the day before and brought it with them. The stuffing, too, prepared ahead of time, so only the vegetables had to be cooked. Mom and Margaret had requested I bring my cheese and asparagus casserole. Their request had surprised me since I hadn't used my oven in months. I'd had instances where I'd forgotten I'd had the oven on and almost burnt the food. The same thing had happened when using the stovetop. I'd stopped using it altogether unless Devon was home. If my sister hadn't known that Mom had. My townhouse wasn't far from Mom's so Dev and I opted to walk over.

We arrived early to spend some time with Mom before the others would arrive later that afternoon. When my sister- and brother-in-law arrived, we gathered in the small living room. It extends the open space with the kitchen near the entrance at one end, and a dining table sandwiched between them. I'd sat cross-legged on the floor next to the coffee table– Mom in her new recliner made of brushed blue velveteen with mahogany arms wrapped in the same material. Margaret and Barry sat on the love seat and Dev on the club chair. I hadn't minded sitting on the floor as I'd been close to the gas fireplace. Ever since my first surgery, I felt cold all the time. My hands frozen and my body chilled even in summer. I'd always had a little furnace burning inside that kept me warm in winter and sweltering in summer. Now, the blankets and throws that would've been folded and put away, are left out and often pulled around me when reading or watching TV–socks and slippers covered frozen toes.

With dinner precooked, we had plenty of time to enjoy drinks and a chinwag. I'd stopped drinking alcohol after that first seizure back in 2015 and opted for ginger ale and cranberry juice while the others enjoyed a glass of wine–or two. The evening was short, and I was thankful for that. I hadn't wanted to hear any more about how many single men were in Calgary and how'd I'd find one. The thing was, I wasn't interested in dating or entering a relationship. I had enough problems dealing with my health. I didn't need the stress of adjusting my life to include someone else. Nor had I wanted to feel the disappointment when I couldn't count on them when I need them the most. I'd had already been there, done that, bought the t-shirts and returned them twice before. I never was much of a shopper, and even less so then and now.

***December 14th, my left hand took on a life of its own***

Thank God for my note-taking, as I don't know how it'd started. I remember something hadn't felt right, and I raced up to my son's bedroom, seeking safety. Being alone during a seizure is uncomfortable and heightens the panic and fear–transports me back to four years ago when this nightmare unravelled my life. Not that I couldn't be alone; it was more about the comfort of someone around me when the beast took over. I'd experienced multiple status events over the previous four months, and the thought of dissolving into the black hole of nothingness was terrifying. We sat on Dev's bed and watched my fingers as they wiggled about like the fluid movements of a squid's tentacles. I was aware of what was happening and asked Dev to video me–provide Edwards and Young with my version of video telemetry–sans electrodes. Clearing out the bookshelf, china cabinet, and TV stand, packing up the contents had thrown my brain into overload. The stress I placed on myself over the remaining months of 2018 was showing. I might've been able to contain it from spilling over, if my mother hadn't taken a spill in the grocery store. It'd happened between Christmas and New Year. The call came through during one of my many Netflix marathons. A number I hadn't recognized flashed across the screen. I ignored it. Figured if it were urgent, they'd call again or leave a message. They had.

"Hello, Linda, it's Dr. Kerry calling. Don't worry, she's fine, but I've got your Mom here in the emergency room. She took a spill and is hoping you'll take her home. Here's my number. I'm in zone two. Give me a callback and let me know when you can head up."

I sat — the familiar rising of panic and fear washed over me. Beating it down below the surface, I returned the call. A brief conversation confirmed she'd tripped and fallen after entering the store. She hit her head. He warned me she looked like hell. She had no broken bones; but she had a swollen eye. I walked the three blocks up to the hospital, oblivious of the cars passing by, the glow of lights shining from the windows of the houses I passed. I met her at the emergency room entrance. She sat in a wheelchair off to the side. She looked frail slouched to one side, head supported on the undamaged side, eyes droopy. I called a cab and took her home. She hadn't called my sister; there wasn't any point. She just wanted to get home. It'd have taken too long for Margaret to drive out from Vancouver while I was only seven minutes away. She swore me to secrecy. Mom would tell my sister in her own time. She sent me home once I'd gotten her settled with water, food, and dressed in a nightgown and robe, which was for the best. Who knew if the stress and overwhelming emotions would have triggered a seizure. The thought of that and leaving Mom by herself had created a flutter of activity in my stomach. My body was torn.

My gut said, 'don't leave' but my head said 'yes, you should go.' My inner battle came to an abrupt halt when she shooed me away. We agreed that I would come back the next morning to check on her.

Her fall had been upsetting, but as the days passed, the left side of her face had turned from her usual rosy complexion to a mottled blue with a hint of yellow-brown, then black. When she'd slipped, she'd hit her head on the edge of a pallet that'd held a display of marked down Christmas items–candies and decorations. Fortunately, she had broken nothing. She just looked like she'd lost her bout in the ring. Considering her accident, I increased my weekly calls by checking in on her. They became so routine you could've recorded our morning conversations and hit the playback button every day. They were that predictable.

Mom: "Morning. How did you sleep?"

Me: "Morning. I slept okay. How about you?"

Mom: "Pretty good, was up again during the night reading. What have you got planned for today? Anything?"

Me: "Not much. Oh, did you see (insert here) in the local paper, any tennis or ice skating on today?" Etc. Etc.

Such had become my life. The daily phone calls with Mom checking in to let each other know we hadn't died during the night.

**Self-reflection**

*As time passed, I withdrew within the circle I'd drawn in the sand: my little island, my hula-hoop. It was my way of trying to take back control. Not one to lie, I censored the information I shared. I'd been a guinea pig and lab rat for so long, I no longer knew the meaning of privacy. Surrounded by doctors and nurses more often than family or friends. In hospitals, doctor offices and shoved in and out of machines. I'd had enough blood drawn to feed an entire vampire family for a week. I craved solitude and peace. I wanted to be alone within my tortured mind - to wander at will. To float in and out, moving as my spirit guided me. I wasn't depressed or lonely. I just needed time alone to get to know myself. To get caught up with the here and now. Tired of living the past few years in constant limbo, I needed to take back my life and for me to do that, my focus had to shift inwards. All outside interferences had to fall away far from the edge of that circle in the sand. I needed to restore my energy levels. I wasn't shutting down; I was preparing to morph into something new. I was about to step outside of my comfort zone; yes, I still had one.*

*While lying in the seizure unit in Foothills, alone, lost and scared, I realized it was there I needed to be. Moving to Calgary had become a seed budding—blossoming into a flower. It would be best for my health and mental wellbeing. I could remove the stress of commuting from BC — the worries of a repeat performance—one without the positive outcome it'd had this time. By remaining in BC, I was exposing myself to potential harm from those who didn't truly understand my disease. The health system hadn't provided the tools to help the thousands of others with Epilepsy that must battle alone to overcome this beast that lives within. The more I thought about it, the more I warmed up to the idea. I could follow in my brother's footsteps and move to the other side of the Rockies. But to accomplish that deed would be far more challenging and complex than I'd expected. For me to choose to sell and pack up to a new city in another province would be unheard of, absolutely impossible if I'd been the old me. Before this, I'd never have entertained leaving my beloved backyard. That person loved the ocean surrounded by white-capped mountains and rolling hills of green and the new me still does, but it came with a cost - my health. Once I decided, excitement took seed and grew. I was eager to take the next left on my travels through life. To wander down roads past cities and towns, forests and lakes I'd never seen or heard of before. Mentally packed and ready to go, the waiting to sell had been the only*

*barrier to crossing the Rockies and I'd hoped, for Susannah's*
*sake, I'd come around those mountains before the snow fell.*

# Chapter Nineteen

## *Same old shit, different year*

On January 3, 2019, I went into status. I was speaking with my cleaner when the fingers of my left hand twitched. My left eye soon followed. Somewhere between a flutter, a wink, and a nervous tic. I'd become familiar with this new form of warning and had called out to Dev. It was fortunate he was home. As it got worse, I had difficulties standing. My legs shook, and I lowered down into a squat as though I were exercising. Dev grabbed my arm and took the brunt of my weight as my legs buckled. In a most undignified manner, my frame collapsed to the floor, all the while twitching, which impeded our progress. He went to grab the Ativan, but it wasn't in its usual spot. I'd put it away as Dr. Young had instructed me not to take it. A lot of my seizures back in the fall felt non-epileptic and the Ativan wouldn't have had any effect. Being addictive, he hadn't wanted me using it to reduce my anxiety and stress. "There are better forms of anti-anxiety medication you could be taking." He'd said.

My cleaner was beside herself — she'd never seen a seizure before and stood off to the side, tears flowing and wringing her hands as she fretted over my welfare - afraid of what she was witnessing. Meanwhile, Dev returned upstairs after his hunt for the Ativan. He told me afterwards how he'd knelt down next to me, cradled my head on his lap, slipped a tablet under my tongue and placed my head onto the pillow he'd brought with him. He talked to me, he said, asked me questions. Questions like, can you hear me? Can you squeeze my hand, open your eyes, or move your legs? At some point, I'd stopped responding and couldn't squeeze his hand. It was then that he called 911.

All of my events had occurred on the second floor of my townhouse. I couldn't tell you the last time I'd been on the main floor when a seizure struck. It would've been far more convenient for the paramedics if they'd occurred on the main floor. The paramedics wouldn't have needed other equipment and more hands to get me into the ambulance. That time, the tractor chair wasn't an option. I couldn't respond to their instructions as I had when guided up out of the belly of my sister's boat. That time they had folded me into a hammock-type sling and they carried me down the stairs to the stretcher and up into the ambulance. I'm sure it couldn't have been easy. I needed a shot of Midazolam on top of the Ativan, and somewhere between home and the hospital, I lost control of my bowels - shitting all over myself. After we arrived at the emergency room, the medics whisked me through triage and deposited me on a bed — a faint memory of being pushed and pulled as they removed my pants and wiped my ass.

[Midazolam is a benzodiazepine medication like Ativan and is used as an emergency treatment for seizures. It's faster acting than other benzodiazepines and is often used alone, or in addition to Ativan.]

**January 22, 2019: Dr. Edwards's follow-up**

After three and a half years, I felt our patient-doctor relationship had become closer than most. To me, he was more of a confidante and close friend. I was an interesting case for him. One that wouldn't come across his desk every day. Unlike some doctors, he was wholly invested in my wellbeing. His devotion to his craft was admirable, almost all-encompassing. Being under his care provided a sense of well-being, as if sitting before a fire, all cozy and warm.

"I know Dr. Young won't like this, but I think it prudent at this point to bump the Lamotrigine back up to 200mg twice a day." That was more than what I'd started at, but less than the toxic amounts pumped into my system the previous year.

"I haven't been as diligent on tracking every little thing like I was. I thought maybe it might be better for me not to focus on what my body is doing every minute of the day. I'm thinking it adds to my stress."

Each month, I'd transfer my daily notes to the calendar. I'd added up the frequency of every wave and anxious/wavy moment. The feelings of light-headedness, almost passing out, and the pains—commented on suspected seizures and unknowns. Every twinge, odd occurrence, words mispronounced or forgotten, altered sleep patterns, and day-to-day activities documented. My heart would sink when the numbers grew or remained constant. I came to dread the tedious task. I tried to joke about it. Referred to myself as Dr. Edwards's freaky patient. It hadn't helped and further down into my well of despair, I'd sank, taking my mind with it.

"I agree. You need not track everything. I want you to continue documenting your seizures and waves. Show those on the calendar. Jot down other things for yourself. Go ahead. All I need is actual seizure-related information."

I nodded and scribbled a note in my book. Placed a star beside it so I'd not forget.

"Oh, yeah. I haven't started my physical therapy sessions for my hand yet. I meet with the therapist on the 30th, so that'll help. Maybe I will see some improvement." I looked at my hand, curling the fingers into a loose fist. The lack of sensation and motor skills had continued to be an issue. The deficiencies hadn't improved over the two months since surgery. Tying shoes, washing dishes, and dropping items I'd forgotten I was holding, had interfered and frustrated my abilities to function. Even to this day, my hand struggles with the simplest of tasks. Opening plastic wrappings and containers–tying and untying shoes–putting on jackets and gloves–folding laundry and making beds. The list keeps growing. That it won't improve only makes it worse. The sensory connection was partially removed—it won't grow back.

My appointment ran longer than the hour allotted. We discussed the feelings I had on my left cheek and upper lip. Areas that felt as though a tiny hair or a bit of fluff had touched the skin, causing me to swipe at my face often. The sensations never occurred on the right, just the screwed up left side. Another mind game to drive me into the ditch. I left his office with a prescription and lab request in hand. With the increase to the Dilantin, he'd wanted to monitor my blood levels. Too high a dose could overload my system making me toxic like I was back in August. Being on six medications had put me in a tailspin. My body couldn't handle all the drugs and reacted by seizing. It wasn't a scenario I wished to repeat. Balancing my Dilantin dosage against the maximum dose allowed while staying within therapeutic ranges had been a challenge for me from the beginning. I've never been within the therapeutic range for optimal effectiveness—it was how my body processed it. The ideal parameters are between forty to eighty, and I'd maintained an average of twenty-five reaching thirty on one occasion. Dr. Edwards instructed me to get the bloodwork completed within the week and return on February 26, 2019, to check-in and go from there.

*** *My Left Hand—What's left of it* ***

I began therapy on my hand at the REDI program operated out of the Community Hospital. I knew where to go as I had been there back in 2015 and 2016 for Cognitive Behaviour Therapy. The ladies in this unit were friendly and helpful. Not every medical professional can have a pleasant, sunny disposition, which is understandable. Faced with ailing patients in pain and feeling at their worst daily is an arduous task. Exposed to grumpy, negative people would wear down most individuals. My experiences with my therapists and unit clerks were anything but negative.

Since my six-hour event last October, followed by the surgery, my left hand had lost a significant amount of agility and a sense of touch. The symptoms were like those of a stroke patient. But it wasn't until I'd almost burnt my hand on a mug of coffee that we realized my deficiencies. When I'd stayed at my brother's after the surgery, my sister-in-law, Carol, had boiled water for our coffee one morning and handed me mine. My hands were chilly, like ice, and had been since the operation. I'd wrapped my left hand around the side while I poured the milk. Several seconds had passed before I'd felt the burn. As the heated mug warmed my hand, a slow burn had become a searing pain. Jesus! Damn, that's hot. I'd just about knocked the mug off the counter when I'd snapped my hand away. The heat of the ceramic had been so severe it could've been a smouldering ember—enough heat to hurt but not to burn.

When I'd gotten home, I'd discovered that cold had the opposite effect. It's like placing my hand through a hole in the ice, plunging it into the icy water below. The reaction was immediate, almost painful. It'd reminded me of when I was a kid, playing in the snow without gloves or mittens–the fingers red and numb–the heat of the indoors burning them as if on fire. Holding onto items such as towels, face cloths, and clothing hadn't registered. My brain wasn't receiving the signal that my fingers were holding onto something. And yet, grasping certain items had hurt as if I held heavy plastic bags–the handles digging into the fingers, leaving red and white lines where it cut the circulation. Just to clean a frying pan was annoying in a different way. The coordination needed to hold it steady with a firm grip while I'd scour with the right proved awkward and sometimes painful. Many a time, it had slipped from my fingers into the sudsy water, splashing me in the face, over the counter and onto the floor. I hadn't the means with which to switch hands. To hold with my right and wipe with the left, switching as fatigue had set in, had no longer been an option. Dropping things had become a regular occurrence. From clothing and towels to cutlery and shoes. To not have the use of a part of your body as you'd had before had been no different from if I'd had a broken arm or a sprained ankle. I consistently adjusted to each situation as they occurred and compensated for the lack of mobility as best I could. It wasn't insurmountable. It was frustrating as hell. Still is. It was apparent my hand wasn't functioning as it should have. We'd discovered that, but what wasn't clear at the time was how much it couldn't do? I wasn't ambidextrous but could use my left hand more so than most. I'd had trained myself years ago to use a computer mouse with my left, freeing up my right to make notes, dial a phone or use a calculator. It'd come in handy when the workload was heavy. I could even hold a paintbrush or roller in both hands. As one tired, the other would take over. Whether broad strokes or touching up trim, either hand had worked well.

***Occupational Therapy–Community Hospital***

At my first session, Michelle, the occupational therapist, had me perform some tests to create a baseline. My first task had been to pick up a handful of marbles one-at-a-time, hold them in my hand without dropping them, and then place them one by one into a bowl. It was slow and tedious, and I lost a few as I went through the exercise. It frustrated me at how difficult it was - a toddler would've done better. She had me run through it several times; the marbles dropping more and more when my strength had weakened. Trying to hold the marbles throughout the exercise, filling the palm one by one, was like placing water in a sieve, expecting it to have stayed. Next had been finger spreading. With my hand laying palm down on the table and fingers together, I was to spread them wide apart and then bring them back, moving them at the same time. Spreading them until I was about to play a piano had been the easier part.

But even then, the muscles and tendons strained as my mind had sent the signals. They hadn't responded at first, and took every effort I possessed to move them. The level of concentration was intense. My focus was unwavering. To close them again was far more challenging. The muscles of my arm twinged, and the tendons plumped up like a hose filled with air as I continued. Michelle asked me to perform the exercise four times, but I only managed it twice. There's a disconnect between my brain and my hand. You just can't cross a bridge when there isn't one. Next up, Michelle placed a board in front of me covered with round pegs the diameter of a small dowel; one side painted white. In a zig-zag pattern, she instructed me to pick up each piece. Turn it over in my hand and without placing it on the table, return it to its place on the board. It, too, shouldn't have been as challenging as it was. The last exercise tested my strength and the lack of sensation. With eyes closed, Michelle handed me objects to describe. She alternated between right and left to determine to what extent they differed. Cups, coins, and whatever object she found around the room she placed into my hands. A travel mug filled with marbles for weight, I'd lift to my mouth and back down to the table. Then I'd lift and place the mug on tables of varying heights, testing my hand's ability to hold it. I saw Michelle twice a week, and the progress was slow. The amount of focus and mental energy I had to tap into was staggering.

329

*[Our brains are a mysterious organ. When functioning as it should, you don't realize how many cells go into operating our bodies. The mind commands every organ, muscle, limb, and thought. When there's a short circuit or the connection breaks, the body goes into shock like a tilted pinball machine. Lights flash, and the flippers stop working. And it cuts power off to protect the main panel from overheating.]*

**Alarm Bells Ringing**

February finished with what I now realize were warning signals. My left hand, the corner of my mouth, and the eye were twitchy, and I'd had a wave and felt off. It'd been like my body and mind were confused and hadn't known which way was which. It was the rumblings of what was to come — a precursor to another storm.

# PART FOUR

## Chapter Twenty

### **A New Home**

*I cried yesterday, For what I lost, for what had been—what will be no more. Memories of the past left behind—fate stole them away. I cried yesterday, Tears of sadness, filled with sorrow, in the darkness—alone. Before the light of morning shines, and melancholy recedes. I cried yesterday, I cried for today—for the tomorrows—for all the yesteryears, I cried.*

The decision to move to Calgary drove my need to get er done. Never one for letting the grass grow under my feet; it was a struggle to learn patience. The pressure I placed on myself to get it together to sell was unreasonable, since I was only a few months post-op. I'd lost muscle mass during my hospital stays, and my brain was still recovering from the bolts screwed to my head that'd held the thirteen electrodes in place and the third resection. Those demands I placed on myself (forced upon) triggered seizures months after. Stress has always been my weakness. It raises my anxiety levels to lofty heights, crashing me down into oblivion. I shut myself off from the world around me. Became a hermit of sorts. What Dr. Everly had said on my last visit was true. I was going through a grieving process - preparing myself to leave this place I called home and all the friends and family I'd been able to lean on for support. That I was in self-preservation mode. I visited places dear to me — the house and neighbourhood where I grew up. Our old house still sat on the corner atop a slopping lawn ending at the lane. The old fir trees we called the kissing cousins gone. They'd grown outside my bedroom window, intertwined as if hugging each other. Birds, squirrels, and even a racoon had peered into my bedroom from the safety of those trees. I visited the restaurants of my youth–a heaviness settling on my shoulders as visions of past dinners and lunches floated through my mind.

I combed the beaches where I'd spent many hours soaking in the sunshine and soothing waves as they caressed the shore, collecting my thoughts. I took pictures to keep those memories alive should mine disappear. Said goodbye to acquaintances and shopkeepers I'd grown fond of over the years. Feelings of sorrow swept over me from time to time. Thoughts of *I'll miss that or them* bubbled to the surface. I lost so much of what my life had been, and there was no going back. I was ready for a new story. The last five years had been a challenge, traumatic, life-changing, and scary as hell. How could it not? I'm not the same person I was before; who would be? Only the propensity to find a positive out of a negative and my warped sense of humour had remained intact. Even after everything I'd been through, I was still here. I joked about some of my worst seizures and had nicknames for the doctors, hospitals, and gadgets. My writing blossomed and grew from just poetry and tidbits to actual stories. Writing had always been my means to cleanse my troubled soul - letting my mind float and drift where it may - flowing down and out my fingertips, decluttering the mind. It was a clearing out of the cobwebs and dusting off old memories tucked away in a corner, hidden but not forgotten. — spring cleaning at its best.

**The Move**

[*To adjust, move forward and grow, I had learned to let go. To control the world around me required energy that had been in limited supply. I had to let the world revolve around me and focus on what was essential to my health and mental well-being. My mantra became: It will happen when it happens, as it should happen. And, Everything happens for a reason, and there's always a reason to when it happens.*]

Moving is one of life's most significant stressors. My energy levels were low, but that didn't stop me from pushing the limits. Buoyed up by the thought of a new chapter of my life, I carried on as if operating at full steam—mistake number one. It didn't take long before the first signs of seizure activity bubbled to the surface. With the added stress, the old feelings surfaced again. The Anxious Wavy sensations, waves, feather-like sensations on my cheek and upper lip, and seeing things. My dribble mouth returned, making eating and drinking difficult again. Preparing the townhouse for listing involved some updating and repairs - some obvious while others cropped up just to frustrate and stress me even further. The living and dining carpet needed replacing. The seam between the two rooms had separated years prior. I hadn't bothered to replace it, had opted to wait until I no longer had to commute to Calgary. It meant looking at samples, bringing them home, getting a quote, and arranging installation. I had to empty the china cabinet, bookshelf, and TV stand, boxing up what would come and disposing of the rest. A lot more work involved than if we hadn't moved. Next on my list was decluttering. I'd not carried around a lot of 'stuff' but Devon was a different species of packrat. Thus, most of the sorting and purging confined to his bedroom, the basement, and boxes labelled as Devon's Keepsakes, Devon's Trains, Videos, Games, etc. He had more boxes squirreled away than me and the kitchen contents combined!

*\*\*March 5, 2019\*\**

It started out innocent enough, then turned into something sinister. I remember the beginning phase and asking Devon to take a video of my movements. Dev had to fill in the blanks and put it all down in an email that I sent to Dr. Edwards with the video attached.

**From:** *Linda McClure*

**Sent:** *March 22, 2019 3:49 PM*

**To:** *Dr. Edwards* **Cc:** *Angela*

**Subject:** *Fwd.: Seizure timeline McClure Linda - March 5,2019 seizure*

*Good afternoon! So. We need to stop meeting like this. You go away. I have a seizure. Stop, rewind, repeat. Lol. Below is Devon's timeline of the event. It wasn't as bad as January's, but still over an hour. · I was putting makeup on · I began having difficulty removing the lid and holding the bottle · The fingers started twitching/moving on their own · I grabbed the Ativan and went to Devon's bedroom · The hand twitching got worse · My left eye and corner of mouth started twitching · My speech became garbled · I recall Dev giving me Ativan twice · To me it felt like one continuous seizure · I vaguely recall him trying to give me a 3rd dose · My memory of the paramedics being taken down the stairs & placed in the ambulance & at the emergency room is foggy · Afterwards, the progress made on my left hand regressed slightly. Motor skills mainly. · More headaches and head pains since · Saw Dr. Everly March 19th and she has changed my Citalopram to Escitalopram. Currently weaning off Citalopram before starting Escitalopram. ·*

*Devon's timeline and video has also been sent to Dr. Young. · Welcome back to the funny farm hahaha*

*Sincerely,*

*Linda McClure*


**From:** *Devon McClure*

**Sent:** *Wednesday, March 13, 2019 5:50:45 AM*

**To:** *Parental Unit (Mother)*

**Subject:** *Seizure timeline*

*From what I recall: 7:00 ish: came into my room saying you are having a seizure with arm shaking. Took a video of it (see attached) 7:03 gave an Ativan, it seemed to help for about 10m. 7:13 seizure started up again 7:18 gave another Ativan. Ativan seemed to help again for about 10 minutes 7:30 ish seizure started up again, and I tried to give a 3rd Ativan but jaw was too clamped 7:33 ish, called 911. 7:40 ish I think? Fire arrived and then I mostly stayed out of my room to give them space. 8:00 ish, ambulance arrived, and you were still seizing a bit 8:15-8:20 ish they take you in ambulance to the Community Hospital. That's what I recall, at least.*


After each seizure, I'd noted how the nerves of my left hand would recoil, affecting my dexterity and had made simple tasks a challenge for me. It'd set me back from the advancements I'd made with my visits to therapy. My stress levels had risen, which had only exacerbated the headaches and nerve pains.

** *March 19, 2019* **

I arrived early at Dr. Everly's office. It'd been almost a year since I'd last seen her. Lots had happened. I brought her up to date on the saga that is my life; and then moved onto the matter at hand, my antidepressant.

"I don't believe I'm depressed so much as anxious. I don't feel like going out and find I'm content to stay at home, writing. I've become a hermit. I don't want to talk to anybody or do anything. Oh, and I read that book; Brain on Fire? And I watched the movie on Netflix. And I've started writing a book."

"Good. I'm glad you did. Your story is unique." She sat in her office chair, one arm slung over the back, legs crossed. Her relaxed posture helped to reduce the tension that'd usually settled in my stomach when I'd visit my doctors—a tightly coiled mass of dread and anxiety.

"So, I wanted to talk to you about changing my medication." There were other drugs I could be on that targeted anxiety. I wasn't depressed, had been more nervous, uptight, and anxious than anything else. A heavy burning lump would settle in my gut whenever I had to go out, or had to be up at a certain time. On those days, I'd wake uber early and couldn't go back to sleep. There I'd be, at 5am, coffee in hand, laptop or Kobo on my lap, sitting on the couch two hours before I'd needed to be. My stomach churning and gurgling away as my mind raced, conjuring up all sorts of mishaps that could've happened and cause me to miss my appointment.

Dr. Everly had been aware of these episodes and how I'd cocooned myself from the world. She explained how my actions and feelings were akin to those grieving. I was going through a mourning process. Distancing myself from friends and family was part of me preparing to leave. It made sense. Born and raised here on the Peninsula, I'd never lived outside of the Lower Mainland. Moving away from everything familiar was a massive undertaking for anyone, let alone one with a chronic disease. When I left her office, I'd wean off of the Citalopram and replace it with Escitalopram. She warned me that the process would be slow. Antidepressants, just like my seizure meds, were not something you could just stop taking without dire results.

That month had been busy with therapy, doctors, and hair appointments. Nothing major to the average joe, however. The heap of projects was growing, and I still hadn't listed yet. The to-do list had progressed, albeit slower than I wanted, when the stove element blew up. Looking back now, it had been comical. I was cooking a frozen pizza when a loud bang and hiss had erupted. My first thought had been the clay pizza tray had broken, dumping the pizza into the element. I pulled open the oven door and peered in. The dish was intact. When I leaned over to get a better view, a tiny flame on the bottom element at the back caught my attention. In a matter of seconds, it went out, but left a glowing ember emanating from the heating element itself. *Now what*? I shut the door, turned the oven off and just stood there. *What do I do? Was it a fire? Do I call 911? No. Who do I call? Anyone?* I grabbed the tablet and Googled the nonemergency number for the fire department.

"Hello. Hi, Sorry to bother you. I'm not sure if this is a cause for concern, but…" I explained to the lady on the other end what had happened. That I was alone and not sure what I should do. She'd said she would send a crew out to check and to keep the oven off. In the past, when the fire truck pulled up out front, I'd been seizing. That time, I greeted them standing up, eyes open, and aware. They pulled out the oven and unplugged

340

it. They checked the breaker for signs of an electrical issue and then informed me my element had blown. That had been the bang. I joked with them about how their visit wasn't my norm; that it was nice to see who was helping me. They informed me there had been no threat of a fire, and instructed me to have the plug checked for damage, then left. I thought to replace it. Thought maybe a new stove would have been a good selling feature. But after discussing my options with my brother, Jim and real estate agent, Marion, I called the repairman. Two days later, the upstairs toilet stopped flushing to the point it almost overflowed. And then followed by the thermostat. The original wire attached to the furnace had given way, creating a short that blown the breaker each time it signalled for heat. Then came the kitchen lights. It started with one. An intermittent flickering, like a strobe without a rhythm. Some days it worked fine, other times we'd not turn them on, relying on the hallway and dining room lights to see by. Then the second light joined in. On and off, they pulsed and flickered as though the switch was flipped on and off repeatedly. I had to call in an electrician. He cut a hole into the ceiling, a new junction box and wiring installed just days before our first open house. It seemed like my home had not wanted to let go. That it had created stumbling blocks to delay the inevitable.

"I've listed today. Know of anybody who wants to buy a townhouse?" I was half-joking. I sat across the desk from Dr. Edwards. Another routine follow-up.

"That's great. When do you think you'll be moving?" Dr. Edwards sat back, getting comfortable. We covered a range of topics, from my health to the medical system. It was like sitting down and catching up with an old friend or a close sibling. "These lightheaded passing out feelings. Can you describe them to me? There doesn't seem to be a pattern to them. I ask because sometimes those symptoms can be signs of something else."

I explained to him my cartoon analogy of seeing stars like Elmer Fudd from Merry Melodies. The feeling of drifting, like a hot-air balloon that shifted as the wind currents changed. Or bobbing out on the ocean as the gentle waves lifted you. I hadn't passed out or fainted. It'd been the *sensation* of those experiences.

"I'm not sure there's any cause for alarm, but to cover all bases…."

"Dot the 'I's' and cross the 'T's'?" I'd interjected, paraphrasing him from the past.

Laughing, he'd replied: "Yes. I want to rule out other possibilities. Let's do a Holter Monitor test. Have you had one before?"

"Yup. Way back in 2012 for that very first seizure."

"I'm going to order it at the Community Hospital and an ultrasound of your heart."

"Okay." He could've said he wanted me to jump out the window, and if it meant it'd help my cause, I would have. Incredible how much power you're willing to give someone when you trust them with your life.

The next day, I had another 'Elmer Fudd' episode. I'd felt off most of the day — a headache that felt like a vice grip squeezing the side of my skull and wavy. My head swam, followed by a powerful wave. My movements and thinking slowed down, lasting 30 minutes or more. That episode differed from the ones before. When the light-headedness, floaty, spinny feelings happened, I'm sitting on the couch - all other functions operating normally. This time it started while standing in the kitchen and carried on even after I'd sat down. *Had it been a seizure?* If it wasn't, the frequency had increased.

I documented it on my calendar to discuss with Dr. Edwards at the next appointment. It was the second episode that week. *Was it stress or the slow progression of introducing the Escitalopram Dr. Everly prescribed? Maybe?* I didn't know for sure and had reached a point where I doubted my ability to differentiate between auras, seizures, and anxiety - questioned everything to do with my seizures.

Throughout that time, I had episodes of seeing and forgetting things. I tried to put milk away in the microwave or a cupboard or going to retrieve it, but not from the fridge. *Was it a sign of old age? Or just distracted?* I had also done something that I'd never had since we'd moved back to the townhouse back in September 2015. That day I'd stood looking at my cat's food dish and wondered where the garbage can was. Our garbage was under the sink where it'd been for the last three and a half years. The spot where I'd stood hadn't hosted a bin since 2010. Nine years ago. I walked straight to that spot from the living room and expected it to be there. A large brown can with a swivel lid we tossed out in 2011 when I'd bought the house with my ex-boyfriend, Daniel. It'd shaken me up. A chill had run through my body, my stomach had knotted up causing a pain deep down inside. *Why did my mind play this cruel trick? Am I losing it? Was this a sign of going insane?* To accidentally go to a cupboard versus the fridge, a drawer versus the pantry, was one thing, I thought. But to go where nothing had stood for years and expecting to find it, spoke to a mind that had been slowly unravelling.

Seizure activity had plateaued over April and May, but all the same sensations remained. My waves continued to crash into the shoreline. The churning g-force-type feelings of anxiousness inside me, followed by thoughts circling in slow-motion, brought me back down to earth disoriented and exhausted. Events of light-headedness increased, and my 'Elmer Fudd' episodes quadrupled. I saw things more often. My cat, splayed out on the floor, or I saw him walk by when he wasn't anywhere nearby. Other times I felt him brush up against my leg, only to find him asleep on his perch by the window. One day, I'd been reading in the living room when, out of the corner of my eye, I'd seen the image of a person walk by. Startled at the thought of someone wandering about, I went to see where they'd gone. But there hadn't been a soul in sight. No one was there. The only movement had been a few leaves that'd rustled along the ground and tree branches waving in the wind. *Had I seen a ghost or heavenly spirit? Maybe.*

Whether these were a case of déjà vu or my mind dredging up images, sensations, and memories of things past, it left me feeling unsettled. To help ease some of my stress, I went to massage therapy. I couldn't remember the last time I'd gone. I thought if I could reduce the tension in my body and loosen the muscles and tendons, I'd see an improvement in my hand. I booked a few sessions. It's a good twenty-five-minute walk each way along quiet streets of family homes and parks. The clinic is in a low-rise building in a strip mall next to a gas station. I could've taken the bus. That was only a seven-minute walk along the trail that led to the high school behind us, through the parking lot, past the soccer and football fields to the bus stop. But I needed the exercise.

Throughout the balance of May and into June, the steady stream of looky-loos petered out. One realtor inquired if I would consider a 'subject to sale' offer. Nope. Not in this market. Such offers dragged on for months as extension after extension was requested. Sorry, Charlie. Bring me an offer with no subjects to sale and then we'll talk. The last thing I needed was to tie myself into something that could go sideways, and I'd be back to where I started. My best option was to sit tight and wait.

When my plan to move was in its plotting stage, there wasn't any competition in sight. Since my listing went up in May, for sale signs popped up, sticking out of the ground like molehills. I ran reconnaissance missions as each unit went on the market. Headphones in place and music playing, I walked to each site. I noted if it had a deck, its location to busy roads and the park. I took pictures and emailed them to my realtor. The competition was growing, and I started to worry.

Frustration, doubt, and fear seeped out of my subconscious. Thoughts of '*What if I don't sell? What if I'm stuck here? How will I manage? I'm not safe here*' whirled around my head—wouldn't listen to the possibility of a positive outcome. I withdrew further, drawing comfort from a tattered and torn security blanket filled with holes.

Yet another open house and no requests for viewing. The radio waves were silent. The stress affected my moods—altered my thoughts. Little things, other people's problems, bellyaching and negativity grated on my nerves. I became irritated when the simplest of things took more effort than usual. 'For *Christ's sake.*' '*Fuck off.*' '*Jeez, Louise.*' were my catchphrases. As the weeks drifted by, the seizure activity increased.

It was after the listing went live that Dev gave up looking for ways to stay in BC. Even with a roommate or two and a second job or better paying one, he just couldn't afford to stay. After weighing the pros and cons, he announced his intentions as only he could.

"So. Mom. I've decided to come with you. I've mulled it over and since I like the cold and snow, and they get w-a-a-ay more thunderstorms than here. Flames are a much better team than the Canucks, and I'll be closer to Uncle Jim and those guys." We were in his bedroom sorting and purging when he declared his intentions. I listened, my mouth twitching as I tried not to laugh.

"Okay. Sounds good to me. As long as you're sure?"

"Yeah. I'm sure. Besides. I need to be there to make sure you don't fall down and die!"

Friday, June 24, 2019: The Holter Monitor was ready for pickup. I was to present myself at the Cardiology department at 8 am. There, they hooked me up to a small piece of equipment that tracked my heart rate. I had one done back in 2012 with a Walkman-type device placed into a large pouch and clipped to my waist for 24 hours. I'd documented movements, such as going to the bathroom, eating, walking, watching TV. It'd been necessary but annoying as I had to remind myself to note my activities–sometimes guessing. Seven years later, technology advanced enough that journaling wasn't necessary. The only instructions given were "don't get it wet." No Fanny Pack this time. It hung from a cord placed around my neck. Far less cumbersome and more comfortable to sleep. I returned it the next morning at 8 am. If my appointment was a week later, we could've cancelled.

# Chapter Twenty-One

## **Have I got a deal for you**

## **Journal Entry June 15, 2019**

*Two open houses and three showings with another tomorrow have not produced any offers, and I'm having to remind myself that it's only been a month and to chill.*

*Patience is not a virtue I possess is not even in my vocabulary. Forcing myself to think positively and wait on the sidelines, hoping to score a deal, wasn't easy.*

*Whether it's the side effects of the escitalopram, the stress or weather changes, I've taken to waking early. Most mornings found me on my laptop, coffee in hand, in the living room, watching the sunrise. Coco took to the early risings, wanting food the minute he heard me stir. It's annoying that sleep past 5am is a thing of the past; however, I've made significant progress on my book. It's beginning to feel real—alive and breathing. What seemed like entries in a journal was now shaping into something more.*

*Focused on selling and writing, I removed myself from those around me. The desire to socialize wasn't there. A new chapter in my book of life was about to be written. New settings, characters and events will unfold on this new journey as I hit the reset button and started over.*

*Looking inward, gauging how I'm feeling, what my body is or isn't doing has been a massive part of my life these last 4 years. I want to go back to how I was 30 years ago. Doing my own thing, by myself without any outside interference. I wish to withdraw from the spotlight step backstage, lurking on the sidelines watching from a distance.*

*I miss the solitude of the peace and comfort of my own company—letting the world go on around me, not having to participate unless I choose to.*

*I was never the centre of attention as a child. Happy and content being alone with no expectations placed upon me. I enjoyed flying under the radar. Moving to Calgary will allow me to go back to recapture the essence of who I am.*

*\*\*June 17, 2019, The Wasp Seizure\*\**

It was weird how it all happened, but that is normal for this disease and especially for me. If I didn't have enough to deal with, wasps moved in under the eaves outback. That day the exterminator came, I felt good. So good, I wanted to run on the treadmill. For some time, I'd felt the urge. When out walking, my steps had quickened almost to the point of a full jog. Mindful of my brain still healing from surgery, I'd kept to a fast walking pace with a minute or two of a slow trot. But that was the day I'd had enough of sitting around. It wasn't doing me any good, as my scale had shown me. So, at 10 am, with exercise gear donned, and trusty iPod in hand, I pushed Start. A steady walking pace to warm up, then building to a gentle jog. It felt so good. So very good. I could've stayed on the treadmill all day but hadn't wanted to push myself. At 53 minutes, I shut it down. I felt great. A warm shower and I was downstairs making lunch. The call came soon afterwards. The exterminator would arrive in half an hour.

I led him from the front door through the living room to the patio door. I didn't follow when he stepped out onto the deck. I showed him the areas while staying tucked out of the way just inside the door, out of sight of the buzzing circle above the sliding door. The mini wasps hadn't only just got up under the eaves, but flitted in and out through a hole in the cedar siding. With his ear up against the opening, he stated he could hear the buzzing on the other side. As he sized up the situation, the comings and goings of these intruders increased. Hazmat suit in place, he began. We chatted through the closed patio door as he worked.

I enjoyed the interaction. My body was still in the afterglow of an invigorating workout. His task now completed, I walked him back through the living room to the door and out to his truck. I recall chatting with him as he discarded his hazmat suit, gloves and loaded up. I waved to my neighbour as I turned to head back in. All I remember is losing my balance as I made my way to the porch. I staggered and tripped over my feet as I made my way, gripping the post before stumbling onto the porch steps. My left leg and arm were not cooperating at all. My equilibrium was out of whack—discombobulated. Somehow, I navigated the four steps, opened both the screen and front doors, and fallen through the doorway into the hall. My grasp on the door handle kept me from tumbling to the floor. Still grasping the handle, trying to steady myself, I yelled up to Dev.

"Dev. I need help. Dev." Lucky for me, it was his day off. Used to my urgent calls for help, he was down the stairs and by my side within seconds. I don't remember seeing him. I was already slipping away. At some point, I couldn't stand any longer. I was in an awkward position, somewhere between a squat and a stretch, and I slipped to the floor.

"I need to sit down." From then on, I faded; only bits and pieces rising to the surface of my consciousness. I don't recall sitting. There's a vague memory of the Ativan placed under my tongue. No clue Dev laid me on my side, a pillow under my head. At some point, Dev administered a second Ativan under my tongue. I'm not sure what occurred next. The 911 call? The third Ativan? I remember asking him to call 911, and I remember the pain in my left arm. The pins and needles escalated to the point my arm and hand were on fire. Bolts of electricity penetrated into every nerve ending under the skin. I recall hearing the sirens — a man talking to me. The paramedic? After that, nothing. As when a movie ends and the credits have rolled by, the screen fades, going dark. My next conscious memory, if you want to call it that, was Devon talking. He was telling someone to cancel my hair appointment scheduled for the next day.

I couldn't tell you when I realized my surroundings or knew what happened. My brain retreated into the fetal position—a defence mechanism against the devastating blows it endured and locking away random points of time. Once the dust settled, and with some gentle coaxing, some missing pieces fell into place. But not all of them. I'd found myself in the ICU, not in the emergency room. A tube pushed up my nose, ECG stickers and cables stuck to my body, and an IV jabbed into my arm. My seizing continued after arriving at the hospital—back-to-back over twenty minutes, even with further medication dumped into my system. I may as well have been in a coma for how doped up I was. Too much a threat to myself, I required close monitoring. That wasn't about to happen in the Emergency room, and they found space in Intensive Care. I've been in a lot of hospitals, and several wards, and undergone every test known to man, but never that bad to warrant a visit to ICU. Guess there's a first time for everything. After three days in the ICU, I was out of danger and deemed fit to go home. They consulted Dr. Edwards and increased my Dilantin dosage up to 400mg, the highest I've ever taken. The hospital faxed over the new prescription to my pharmacy, which was great, but the only thing was, all my meds had been in blister packs. It meant Devon had to go home, grab them, take them up for a change, and then go back. The pharmacy spared him the return trip and dispatched them later that day to home.

Fate intervened. A young couple returned for a third viewing. Their offer to purchase came the next day. The powers that be took sympathy on me and offered their helping hand. I was out walking when my realtor, Marion, called with their terms. It was the first of many. Stop. Start. Stop. I'd get only a few yards in between Marion's texts. They'd offer, then I'd counter. Back and forth we went. I abandoned my outing and headed home. By that evening, we struck a deal. I accepted an offer with some minor subjects and a removal date in a week. *Hallelujah. 'May the Saints be praised.'* With fingers and toes crossed, in five weeks, we're gone.

Lists formed in my mind. Contact my mover. Arrange for packers. Get the cat to the vet for updated shots and check-up. Open a cash account. Find a lawyer. See if the buyer wants the TV stand. Arrange for cleaners. Sort through storeroom. As per my norm, the list kept growing. As random thoughts popped up, new items were added. A tickertape a mile-long spewing out of control. I had to pull the plug before it grew and overwhelmed me.

*\*\*Things Ramp Up\*\**

[I was a shadow that lurked in the darkness. A presence felt, but not seen. My spirit almost extinguished. I was a shadow of my former self, fading in and out as if the connection had broken— was intermittent. Now a stranger unsure of who I am and what I wished to be; my identity is unknown. I'm lost in the shadows of fear on a journey to nowhere.]

The anxious wavy periods and light-headedness, plus nausea and confused moments, occurred daily. My mind continued to play tricks on me, having fun at my expense. The left hand hadn't returned to the status quo since the June status event hovering somewhere between before and after. I had almost given up on the hope of selling and resigned myself to remaining stuck in a city within a province that offered me no help. That I'd had no future and no control over this disease that ruled over my body. It took away the inner light that once lived within me.

*\*\*Beginnings—Of Hope—July 8, 2019\*\**

The first time I'd heard about intravenous immunoglobulin (IVIG) for autoimmune epilepsy was during my phone appointment with Dr. Young. Autoimmune epilepsy is a recent discovery over the last decade. Only a few cases diagnosed and they have conducted very little research over the last decade. The IVIG treatment would involve administering a sterile solution of concentrated antibodies alternated with a steroid such as Prednisone into my vein to bolster the immune system. As I understood it, the antibodies attack the neurons, which causes the seizing. Even though all of my tests for autoimmune diseases were negative, it was possible that I'd had a type not yet discovered. It was the only thing left that we hadn't tried. With my epilepsy progressing, Dr. Young felt we should give it a try. I became a guinea pig again.

# Chapter Twenty-Two

## **Just before you go**

*****August 6, 2019*****

It strikes again, my enemy from within, that struggles to overtake my body to get out. After running errands and visiting with Mom, I deposited myself on the couch to watch Netflix. I was on the 2nd episode of Star Trek when I'd felt its presence. Pre-empted by the lost in space and light-headedness, I sat in a stunned-like position for 5 to 10 minutes, maybe less. It progressed to a rushing feeling as if I were about to pass out. My left hand exploded with surges of electrical type shocks radiating up the forearm. It ebbed and flowed - advanced, then retreated. It sprung to life as my mind and body fuelled the flames before settling down to a slow burn. Devon had not yet arrived home from work, and so I self-administered one Ativan. It was the early stages of the seizure, and the one dose should have been enough. But it wasn't. Minutes later, before Devon arrived home, my speech became slurred, and I struggled to find words–had been harder yet to get them out. Moments later, Dev burst through the door, not bothering to close it. He rushed to the couch, dumping his bag in the hall. Kneeling, he glanced at my face, the position of my body, and checked for any movement.

"Can you squeeze my hand?" He asked, lifting my right hand from my lap. "Look at me." He instructed. "Sup. Can you speak? Say something." He turned to the coffee table, grabbed the bottle of Ativan and administered the 2nd dose under my tongue. By that point, I wasn't responding. I hadn't moved, couldn't talk, to have kept my eyes open was impossible.

"911. What's your emergency?" The operator answered.

"Ambulance. My Mom is having a seizure." Devon responded. He'd gone on and answered the questions thrown at him in rapid succession. "Yes, she's already had two Ativan and is not responding. Yes, she's breathing. Yes, sorry? I can't hear you. Hello? Yeah, her phone is crappy. Call me back on mine." My phone was experiencing connection issues, which we'd been investigating. Then wasn't the time for it to act up.

"Yes, no change. Still no response. Yes, there's a family history. She's on medication. Let me get her card. She's on Dilantin, Lamotrigine, Escitalopram, Mometasone, and some other eye drop stuff. Yeah, the fire truck is pulling up. K. Bye."

I heard what went on around me. If my eyes could've remained open, I'd been able to see the faces of my rescuers. They transferred me from the couch to the floor, resuming their examination until the ambulance arrived. The vortex engulfed me, commandeered my brain, and I struggled to stay afloat. The Ativan kicked in enough and allowed my subconscious to surface. Exhausted by the strain and over-medicated, my thought processes were slow to return. If I didn't have epilepsy and a healthy heart, you could've said I'd had a stroke. I spent four hours in the emergency room, had an ECG, a visit from the in-house vampire, and returned to my son's care dopey, weak, and depleted of all energy. Devon helped me move from the wheelchair to the backseat of a cab. By the time we arrived home, I was starving. I hadn't eaten dinner, hadn't had any nourishment since lunchtime. I couldn't bother to eat and went to bed hungry, tired, and sore.

**August 11, 2019**

My last appointment with Dr. Edwards was on August 12. Almost four years to the day since he walked into my hospital room. I awoke on the 11th, tired from another night of intermittent sleep. I was still waking early, regardless of what

361

time I crawled into bed. It was reminiscent of the months leading up to the 2015 seizure, which set me on this wild and crazy ride. By late morning, the signs showed. I saw things, and the side of my head hurt as if whacked with a blunt object. The lightheaded, dizzy sensations took over—my 'Elmer Fudd' interpretation after a hit to the noggin. I was on my laptop, and as my state altered, my typing deteriorated as my left hand refused to hit the keys as directed. Minutes or seconds ticked by; I don't know how long when the pressure built. The walls of my brain felt stretched, as though they were going to snap. My head was imploding, or so it seemed to me. At some point, I grabbed my Ativan and brought it to the couch where I sat. I was on my own and sought the safety of a soft landing pad should I lose consciousness. Devon had gone over to a friend's the night before and hadn't yet returned. It was me, myself, and I for this one. I messaged him to let him know, and that I was taking an Ativan. I needed to reach out to someone. Licking my lips and rubbing my palms on my thighs, glancing at my phone and away, then back again, I grabbed it, took a deep breath and began typing. I hadn't wanted to spoil his fun with his friends; he may not see them again before we left. My tormentor knew his time was running out, and with a last push, a wave hit–short but hard. Eight minutes after taking my dose, the monster crept back into the shadows. It passed, and I carried on with my day. Picked myself up, dusted off and walked away. Like a ballplayer who slid across home tying up the game. Throughout it all, besides wishing it to go away, I feared it would escalate. *I can't go to the hospital. I have to see Dr. Edwards tomorrow. Please don't do this to me. Hold on until I get to Calgary. You can take over and have at er once I'm there.*

**Goodbye White Knight**

*August 12, 2019,* I was up by 5am still tired but unable to fall back to sleep. I've always enjoyed my visits with Dr. Edwards. It was like visiting an old friend who meted out expert advice. Angela booked me as his last patient of the day.

"So, you sold. That's fantastic. Especially with this market. Some houses are taking forever to sell."

"Yeah, thank God. I sold to a nice young couple with two little kids. I didn't get as much as I thought, but I am pleased with what I got. How was your vacation?"

"It was terrific. We enjoyed it. But as you know, it's hard to come back after being away." We settled ourselves across the desk from each other.

"Yeah, you work your ass off to get ready to go and then have to catch up when you're back."

"When do you leave?"

"In ten days. That's it, and we're gone. Leave on the 22$^{nd}$."

"You're going to be in expert hands. Dr. Young and the team will look after you."

"I know, but it means leaving you. It's been four years since we met, on my 50$^{th}$ birthday, you know."

"Yes, I know."

"Where did that time go?"

"Is it going to be hard leaving? Are you going to miss it here?"

"You know. It's not so much missing the physical. I mean, I was born and raised here and loved the water, but it's the people I'm going to miss more. Funny thing is, I'm going to miss my doctors more than my friends."

"Yes. It's amazing how close we can get to our doctors when fighting an illness."

"So, I had another seizure. Not as bad as the others. They only kept me overnight. No, wait, sorry. I stayed only a few hours. Oh, and I had another one yesterday. Only mild, though." I explained what had occurred the day before. My mind was empty of the events earlier in the month. I confused my last seizure with the one in June when admitted into the ICU. I was missing chapters out of a book, interrupting the flow of the story. We moved onto how I was doing at that moment: the frequency of waves, the situation with my left hand and arm, my balance issues, etc.

"How often would you say the waves are happening? Have they increased or decreased?"

"I think they're the same. Or maybe less. I see things more, though. And my left hand hasn't been all tingly and pins and needles like it was. Since the last seizure, I've had days where there weren't any. But then, like with that seizure when I said my left arm hurt? It'll come back—intense. Pulsating, nerves vibrating. Flares up and recedes, like flames in a fire, you know?" He sat across from me, listening intently. And I knew he was, you could tell by looking in his eyes. They weren't all glassed over with a vacant stare as his patient rambled on about their symptoms. "I'm wondering if when the intensity increases in my arm if it's seizure related? The pin and needle thing is pretty much constant, but when it flares up, it's when a seizure hits. There was that big seizure at the beginning of that week I had my surgery. It affected my hand and then after the surgery…" My voice trailed off. He knew the rest.

"I'm not sure the arm is seizure-related. But Sam and his team will figure that out. That's why I did that MRI of neck and shoulders earlier in the year; see if there was something like a pinched nerve. The arm is definitely because of the surgery, but it should get better, not worse."

"On my last call with Dr. Young, he talked about trying immune therapy or steroids as a next step. Can't keep drilling holes in my head."

"No, no, they can't. Yes, that would be a logical step, I agree."

"So, I know he explained it to me, but you only have so much time when on the phone. What does this involve? Do I stay in the hospital?"

"No, done at home, you know, as an outpatient. When we were trying to figure out the cause of your seizures, we tested for autoimmune diseases. Remember? We tested here twice, and Calgary did too. We looked for NMDA and others, but you tested clean. By doing immune therapy, we can trigger antibodies that aren't showing on test results. It's a possibility you may have one they haven't discovered yet."

"Okay, that makes sense. Hey, I could have one named after me." We laughed.

As he settled back to his position across the desk, my head spun. It felt floaty, like a balloon wafting in a breeze.

"I-I'm having one of my waves..." My voice trailed off as the rush washed over me. The room froze, yet I wasn't immobile. A vibration deep below had risen, expanding across each nerve. It only lasted a moment, then receded.

"Are you with us again, Linda?"

"Uh, yeah. It's gone now." We continued our conversation as though nothing happened. This event wasn't anything new to either of us. Seen many others before, and after four years, they became as normal to me as breathing- sometimes.

"Could I be having mini-strokes?"

"No, they wouldn't manifest themselves in this manner."

"I've noticed that, um, I've been 'umming' a lot again. Having trouble searching, finding words and such."

"You seem and sound fine to me. Your speech, how you're talking, has improved from before."

"It's gotten worse again with all these seizures. Like my hand, it's regressed somewhat. It depends on how much or how often during the day I've been talking. I spend a lot of time alone, so could that make a difference? I have no problems coming up with conversations by myself. The words flow with ease from my head to the keyboard." We laughed. It was true. I had a far easier time conversing through my fingers than via my mouth.

"Well, that makes sense, but you have improved." We chatted some more—tears dripping down my cheeks. I knew I was going to cry.

"I'm going to miss you guys."

"We're going to miss you, too. I'm going to miss you. With all that you've endured, you've handled it with grace and style. It can't have been easy."

It was time to end our last meeting together. I gathered up my stuff.

Standing, the doctor said, "Now I'm going to hug you."

"Good, cause I was going to hug you." In a tight bear hug, patting each other on the back, we said goodbye.

"I'm going to miss you. Keep in touch, eh?"

"I'm going to miss you, too." He had phone calls to make. He placed his 'Administrator's Hat' on as I left. I never thought it would hit as hard as it did. I walked through the doorway down to the elevator; *this is the last time I'll be doing this.* My heart was heavy. I felt like I was going to a funeral or walking the last mile before the light snuffs out. Taking a deep breath, I pushed the button down the elevator into the lobby.

"Taxi."

"Hi, how are you today? Can you send a cab?" And that was that.

# Chapter Twenty-Three

## **Are We There Yet?**

The gym equipment wasn't packed up, my freezer still sat in the laundry room, and no takers for the glass-topped coffee table.

"I'll take the table and place it on the side of the road at my place if it comes to it," my friend Janine offered. The scattered pieces started forming together to complete the final picture. The week started rocky. The seizure on Sunday, my friend not coming for the freezer as promised, and I still had to find someone to pack up our gym equipment.

In desperation, I called my mover, and she arranged for their guy to come on Friday, August 16th, to dismantle and pack up the equipment.

Life plays tricks on us. Taunts and teases us just for laughs. I found myself back on the 6th floor where I was the year before, two weeks shy of the day. I planned to spend the weekend doing nothing to conserve my energy for the shit show of a week looming before me. I was racing about almost in a panic, trying to finish up the few many to-do's. The last task for the day was to dismantle the treadmill for Wednesday's shipment to Red Deer. I was passing it on to my brother. Margaret gave it to me when she retired in 2017 and I was handing it over to our brother, Jim. Through our mover, we hired a tech to dismantle and pack it and the weights for shipment to Jim. The tech hadn't finished before my brain went into overdrive. Standing in the kitchen, I became woozy and lightheaded.

"Go sit down, Mom," Dev said once I'd told him. I moved to the chair and sat sideways, leaning to one side. My arm wrapped around the back, resting on a rung of the back. I sank into my world. My body became limp like a Raggedy Ann doll. It forced Devon to push and pull me so I wouldn't fall from my perch. I was too heavy for him to move me to the floor. Ativan hadn't stopped it and another 911 call made. Like last time, I heard what was going on around me, but responding was an issue. I couldn't keep my eyes open for much more than a moment or two. Talking was out of the question. My bones may as well have been mushy pulp; my muscles overstretched elastic bands.

"Linda, keep your eyes open. Open your eyes, Linda." The medics attending to me repeated over and over. One pinched my left shoulder to gain a response. Then jabbed his fingers into the flesh and muscle at the base of my neck. The pain was like nothing I've felt before. Excruciating. While it registered and my eyes opened, no sound escaped my lips, my internal screams unheard. In the ambulance, they abandoned their attempts to start an IV. Once in the emergency, they'd tried again but failed. My mouth started twitching and still without an IV. The nurses scrambled and eventually succeeded. I awoke in a room. The clock said it was after 4. Even with my fuzzy head, I knew it was 4 am not pm. My seizure started around 5 or 6 pm the night before, that much I knew. The doctor saw me later that morning. He looked young. Clean shaven with blond hair cropped short, he appeared no older than a freshman in college. I wondered just how much experience he had. He sat in a chair and reviewed the previous day's events, concerned that it was my third seizure that month; he wanted to keep me over the weekend.

"I'm moving to Calgary. I've got packers coming and two different shipments going out this week. We leave on the 22nd,

I have things to do and appointments to keep. I can't stay." I ran out of breath in my need to convince him to discharge me.

"Ms. McClure, I realize that, but we're conducting other investigations. We need those results before you can leave. If all goes well, and you have no seizures, you could head home in 24 to 48 hours." He stood to leave as he spoke.

"What kinds of investigations?" *What is he talking about? I had a seizure, and bloodwork completed on Tuesday, for Christ's sake?*

"We're looking for signs of infections and other causes." He stated as he walked towards the door.

"Are you serious? Do you realize that you're causing me more stress by keeping here than if you sent me home? You're increasing my chances of another seizure." It had been at least ten hours since my seizure stopped and no activity since. It was a prolonged status event, but nowhere near the intensity of the August 6th one, and they sent me home the same day. In the past, once conscious, and able to drink, talk, walk, and go to the bathroom, they released me. I could see keeping me overnight. This time, I was pretty doped up but felt fine other than the residual Ativan hangover. I was eating, drinking, talking, walking, and going to the bathroom by myself; there was no need to keep me.

"Like I said. We will wait and if all goes well, you can go on Sunday." With that, he strode out of the room.

I was tired, as was normal after events such as these. I hadn't been sleeping well, and my mind was in race mode, trying to get everything done before the packers arrived. I planned to spend the weekend with my feet up, doing nothing. As much as I wanted to go home, it was in my best interest to stay one more day. I resigned myself to remain a temporary, unwilling captive. Tomorrow, I had other plans. I was breaking out regardless of the doctor's orders and would sign the docs to secure my freedom come hell or high water. When informed that the on-call neurologist was increasing my Dilantin, it outraged me. *How can a specialist provide a recommendation without seeing the patient? A doctor who's never seen me before?* Dr. Edwards just increased my dose. And I explained my Epileptologist in Calgary did not want my dosages to increase. I was here last year because I was toxic, and he didn't want a repeat of that. They did not care. This mysterious neurologist felt piling on more medication was the answer. To placate me, the nurse said he was to visit another patient on my ward that day and might pop by. I don't know if he saw that other patient, but he never came to see me. I wasn't impressed with the neurologists at Sullivan or Community, apart from Dr. Terry and Edwards. Out of five stays in the hospital, I'd seen a neurologist once and handed a prescription four out of the five times. Doctors backed away from my case as I was declared too complicated. "Too many cooks in the kitchen," according to one. "Guess this is her new normal," stated another. I'm just *one speck of sand along the West Coast, insignificant, unimportant.*

Another uneventful day and night. I prepared myself to fight the establishment and sign myself out. But I didn't have to. The bed manager arrived to discuss my pending discharge, and I regaled her with my tale of woe.

"I'll leave a message for the doctor and let him know your intentions. If he wants to be part of it, he can come to see you."

Sometimes digging in your heels nets the desired results. He arrived soon after and agreed to release me. The nurse handed me my prescription—based on the neurologist's thorough examination of my situation. And a copy of the Discharge report.

# Chapter Twenty-Four

## *Please Fasten Your Seatbelts and Remain Seated***

Our last day was busy and long. The movers packed our belongings the day before and returned around 9 am the next morning to load up what was going into storage in Calgary until we found a place. Up early, we had all the last-minute to-dos completed before they arrived. Our realtor and long-time friend Marion arrived with breakfast and to grab the Shaw equipment, she'd return for us. Mom showed up soon after. We had to leave for the airport by 2 pm, and if the movers hadn't finished, she would stay behind to complete the paperwork on my behalf. It wasn't necessary. The movers finished with time to spare. While Dev and I waited for our ride to the airport, we said our goodbyes. Mom had called a cab to take her home. Her knees could no longer handle the fifteen-minute walk. We hugged and kissed as her ride pulled up. She wore a brave face; but couldn't stop the tears welling up and a slight quiver of lips before she took her seat. All settled and buckled in; she headed off. The guilt of leaving her sat heavy on me.

Margaret lived in Vancouver, which left Mom without the convenience of a family member a mere ten minutes away. Dev had worked at the mall across from her building, and was there to pick up groceries and provide much-needed tech services, and pop in for visits. It felt as if I had abandoned her.

The van I booked to take us to the airport provided ample space for the two suitcases, carry-on, laptops, our cat, Coco's crate, and Dev and me. Coco surprised us with how calm he was. None of his usual meowing and caterwauling erupted from within his confined space. Even at the airport, when asked to remove him from the crate, he did not panic — my worries of how he'd manage were unfounded. They took him away to a holding area where other pets were waiting for loading. We didn't see him again until we arrived in Calgary. Seated and strapped in, carry on, and personal items stowed, I felt a wave rumbling up from the depths. I was tired and stressed and overstimulated. The last thing I needed was to seize on the plane 10,000 feet up. I turned to Dev. "I'm feeling a bit off, so I'm taking an Ativan. In case."

The flight was uneventful. Coco's first plane ride didn't seem to phase him, which was an immense relief. My overactive mind had visions of finding him panicked or half dead. It had been a long day, and with the time difference, I felt drained. "We're here, Dev. We made it."

My friend Chris picked us up at the airport. We would stay with her and her hubby Jerry until Jim finished his basement and we could head up to Red Deer. Her two cats could've posed an issue, and the thought of Coco banished to a kennel had been a foregone conclusion, but our concerns were unfounded: the cats tolerated his presence, and all was fine. I fell into bed that night and slept right through. But Devon had been sick in the early morning hours. A flu-like bug had invaded his space, and he was up most of the night. The unfortunate thing felt like shit the next day. Fortunately, his recovery hadn't taken long, and he could come out for a ride the following day. I'd wanted to look around downtown at two apartment buildings I'd considered for our new home.

*\*\*Welcome Back August 25, 2019\*\**

*[How much longer could I go on? How long before whatever strength that remained would give way? How much time left before I gave in? Before raising the white flag, admitting defeat?]*

I knew I would end up back in Foothills and the SMU, but didn't think it would occur as soon as it had. We arrived in Calgary on the 22nd and in the wee hours of the 25th; I returned to my home away from home.

Tired after our drive around the city and a trip to Walmart for groceries, I'd gone to bed early. But my stomach had other plans. An hour after taking my evening meds, I was leaning over the kitchen counter, head in the sink. Wiped out, I had no trouble falling asleep. It was dark still when I got out of bed. As I exited my room into the hallway, my hand became numb and twitchy, and then I stumbled. I yelled out to Chris that I needed help. I crashed down the hallway towards her room, banging into the closet doors. I remember sitting on my bed, Chris beside me while Jerry ran to wake Dev. The Ativan appeared and deposited under my tongue. When I came to, I was in a room on the 11th floor—my old stomping grounds at Foothills. It'd been my 3rd seizure in less than a month.

I remained for a week. My Dilantin increased another 50mg to stabilize me. Dr. Kennedy, the neurologist on duty, had wanted to keep the increased dose and discharge me once satisfied I wouldn't have another occurrence. I was adamant he consult with Dr. Young. I'd refused to have my dosages increased, or another drug added to avoid a repeat of the previous summer. Dr. Young's instructions to me had been clear. We had to keep my meds down to prevent toxicity. If we kept bumping them up or adding more drugs, I would become a zombie again. Dr. Young was away and wasn't back until the next week, so I had to wait. Dr. Kennedy entered my room with some news. He spoke with Dr. Young and, if I was willing, I could start the IVIG therapy. I recalled Dr. Young and I had discussed this earlier in the year, and I opted to stay for the procedure. A course of steroids followed by antibodies via IV alternating throughout the day for five days. As Dr. Kennedy explained, the theory behind the treatment was to determine if I had a rare form of epilepsy—Immune epilepsy. Immune epilepsy has only been a concept within the last ten years. The research is limited and has only a few undergone testing. My understanding was one's antibodies attack the neurons in the brain, which then triggers the seizures. Once again, I played the role of guinea pig. They knew I was a willing participant and had no hesitation in approaching me.

"You know, when I speak with Dr. Young about patients, I have to go over their case details to bring him up to speed. With you, all I had to do was mentioned your name."

*[No one likes to feel like they don't exist. But remembered by a doctor busy as Young? That's somewhat 'daunting.' I considered myself blessed to have him thanks to Terry and Edwards. Terry led me to Edwards, who handed me over to Young. Terry, my grumpy old teddy bear. Edwards, my white knight, and Young, my lifesaver, brought me through this to where I am today — starting a new chapter in a new city, a different province.]*

The treatment went well, and with no adverse side effects. Discharged after five days, I left with yet another batch of prescriptions. As part of the therapy, I was to continue with the steroid Prednisone. In addition, they instructed me to take vitamin D and calcium and another drug for my stomach to counteract the effects of the steroid. My seizures had been occurring every month, so it wouldn't be for three to four months of seizure freedom before we have considered it a success. It failed.

**September 2, 2019 Honey, I'm home**

I was getting antsy. Without my treadmill and not getting out and walking, the desire to don my runners was consuming me. Right across the street was a bicycle path that stretched north and south as far as the eye could see. Off I went, music playing and a fanny pack around my waist, carrying ID, Ativan, a list of medication, and my phone. I've learned to have these with me in case of a seizure. My medical alert necklace only told paramedics I had epilepsy, nothing else. It was exhilarating to be out in the fresh air. Heart rate elevated, blood pumping, muscles working, and listening to tunes, letting my mind wander, free of worries. I walked to the south, turned around, and headed back. The confusion must have hit as I headed north. I walked right past the house. I saw a white picket fence. *That's where I need to go.* Somehow, I left the path and wandered off down unfamiliar streets, not knowing where or how I got there. I stood looking up at the signs. Pulling out my phone, I sent Chris a text. I'm lost, lol. I'm at the intersection of Lynnview and Lynnview Way. At some point, I turned down the street, ending up at a house. My left hand started tingling, worsening at each step.

A seizure was starting, and I needed to sit down. I walked up to the nearest house and sat down on the front steps. I wasn't able to open my Ativan bottle; I panicked. I need help. The front door flew open as I banged on it, yelling, "Help! I need help. I'm having a seizure." The fellow was pleasant and tried to understand what was happening. A neighbour who witnessed the drama came over to help. Between the two of them, they sat me down, asked me where I lived, and helped me administer an Ativan. Someone called 911, and Dev and Chris showed up as the ambulance arrived.

In the emergency room, more seizures and Ativan followed. Admitted and sent back up to the 11th floor, where the next day, they put me into the SMU–my fifth visit. After ten days and five seizures, they set me free. None of them had registered on the EEG, so we'd come full circle back to a diagnosis of non-epileptic seizures (PNES). It'd been a relief, sort of. Therapy treats them, not drugs, and I could now access specialists who would help me. On an emotional level, I felt guilty. *Am I so lonely? I'm faking them, seeking ways to get attention and wasting everybody's time?* So many thoughts ran willy nilly through my mind and I had no control, no way to stop them. Much later, we discovered my text went to my sister, not Chris. It was a garbled mess and resembled nothing like what I thought I typed. It said: *Lynnview eau an road intersection.*

*\*\*Journal entry September 3, 2019\*\**

*I found myself back in the emergency. Another seizure. I didn't remain on the neurological ward. Drs Norris and Ivy moved me into the seizure unit, hooking me up to EEG. It wasn't long before the twitching started and I pressed the event button alerting the nurse.*

*"What's going on Linda?"*

*"I-i—i-mm-m-m tw-t-wit—i-it-w-tch-ch-n-n-n-g-g."*

*"Yes, I can see that. Can you tell me your name?"*

384

*"Li-li—i-nn—d-d-a-a Mmcc—m-mc-c-l-u-rrr-r clr."*

*"Good. Where are we?"*

*"F-ff-ff-ot-t f-foot-t-t h-hi-h-h-i-il-lll-sss."* Talking during these events was difficult. The words were all there. It was just getting them out of a mouth that refused to work. No injection this time. A 1 milligram tablet of Ativan under the tongue settled things down.

*My epilepsy is resistant to drugs and has posed a challenge. Have the surgeries opened a gateway which allowed this disease to spread? What about these non-epileptic seizures they believe are a part of the picture? Will some simple therapy harness them? And what about this latest thought of a rare immune epilepsy? Is that the culprit? The bad seed which escaped detection, or is this just a figment of an overactive mind capable of creating make-believe scenarios that would make Spielberg jealous? Will we ever figure this out and bring some balance to my life? There comes a time where you start to question your sanity. Am I causing this, making it happen on purpose as some perverse way of gaining attention? To stand in the spotlight when looking in from the shadows had been sufficient before? Is this my lot in life?*

*So far, this move has not provided the peace of mind I had envisioned. My arrival into Foothills by ambulance twice, finding myself back in a 9 by 9 cell on candid camera performing like a circus monkey for doctors. I am safe here more so than anywhere else, but the walls circle me and my tether keeps me from escaping. I was looking forward to apartment hunting this week, getting to know the transit system and downtown core, shopping for new furniture. I wanted to create a new nest of my own, super cozy and comfortable. My sanctuary in a world that barely knows I exist, outside of Foothills, that is.*

*I've had episodes which haven't shown up on EEG and we're exploring the non-epileptic angle again. I feel guilty, as if I'm causing these unnecessarily. Am I faking them, or are they real? I can't help but think I'm taking time away from others whose need is far greater. That I'm wasting everyone's time and haven't warranted all the time and money they've invested in me. What about family and friends and all the pain and worry I've caused them? The guilt sits like a rock in the pit of my stomach.*

*\*\*Journal entry September 10, 2019\*\**

*This isn't the first time this PNES diagnosis has been brought up during my visits. June 2017 and September 2018 showed the same hypothesis until the depth probes were inserted. Then, it was determined the majority of events were caused by my epilepsy. For the PNES therapy, BC hadn't the resources available and a decision was made not to find a suitable alternative. The events were few and far between and, therefore, seemed manageable. Sitting here now I look back and wonder: should've, could've, would've. If I'd made more effort seeking out some form of therapy, would it have made a difference? Could I have avoided this fifth visit to the SMU? Possibly developed techniques to avoid the emotional turmoil that triggers them. Maybe the third surgery, selling my home and moving, may have been avoided. The worst part of the PNES is they're treatable. I can control them, so why can't I? The guilt that comes after each subsequent seizure is growing, and I blame myself for letting them occur. It's my fault. It's a put on. A bid for attention. I let them happen without a care for how those close to me are affected. I'm wasting the time and resources of the doctors, nurses, labs, hospitals, and ambulances.*

*I don't deserve to be here.*

*\*\*The Verdict\*\**

*The verdict is in. My recent seizures <u>are</u> non-epileptic in nature. If I had epileptic ones, they're too hard to discern and not much can be done. I'll continue to have them. Therapy with a professional specializing in diagnosing the cause of my non-epileptic events can drastically reduce and possibly eliminate them. I've had all the surgeries my brain can handle and while I've been on a combination of most of the drugs, there are some we have not tried and there's the hope of new and improved medications in the future. Once my subconscious mind has been calmed, I can move forward. A new life and fresh surroundings should give me the power to reclaim some of my independence and free spirit, my old self which has been buried by fear, anxiety, and the adverse effects of my medications. I will grow and blossom when I get back to the person I was before this journey began. But it won't be the same. My experiences these last four and a half years have changed me. I'm not that person anymore.*

*\*\*Journal entry—September 11, 2019\*\**

- *Non-epileptic seizures are longer than epileptic.*

- *But. I have long epileptic seizures to begin with, so will be difficult to ascertain.*
- *Ativan won't do anything for non-epileptic seizures. No point taking for these. Only call 911 if really not sure.*
- *Epileptic seizures include confusion, not knowing where you are, slow to respond and don't include the jerking.*
- *Leaving meds alone for now, possibly change up mix if epileptic ones continue.*
- *Not much else can be done as already had all there is.*
- *Treating non-epileptic via therapy will deal with whatever is going on in subconscious that I'm not aware of.*
- ***This is a good thing!!*.*

*\*\*September 25, 2019–Hello Again\*\**

"Hello, Ms. McClure." Dr. Young entered the exam room and squeezed my hand as he closed the door. "I hear you've moved. That's good. I'm glad."

"Dr. Young, after all these years, you can call me Linda." Smiling up at him, I squeezed his hand back.

"So. What's been going on?" I looked at him across the desk, amazed at how relaxed he was. He'd lost weight, had a healthy tan, and didn't carry that stressed, overworked; I'm taking on the world appearance. He looked terrific. I reintroduced my son, and we began reviewing my tales of woe–My introduction to 'Alberta life'–how I spent the first two weeks in the hospital.

"You are an enigma." He'd stated with a ghost of a smile. "But the good news is, if you look at it that way, is the recent seizures were non epileptic. You know, it's not uncommon to have both epileptic and non-epileptic seizures. The treatment options are different." As he spoke, he relaxed back into the chair, raising his arms up and behind his head. I stared in wonder, as he'd never done that before. Was always the professional, a stickler for formality; had never shown this side of him.

"I know. It's good and bad. I mean, it's good to hear it wasn't my epileptic ones. But it's like I'm faking it and wasting everybody's time; the doctors, nurses, ambulance..." Tears filled the corners of my eyes. My chest constricted as I'd fought to keep a lid on my emotions.

"Yes, that's normal to feel like that. But it's not your fault. Your brain can only handle so much. You may have something going on within which you have no concept of–a trigger you don't even know exists." Reaching across the desk, he patted my hands — an intimate touch. One meant to comfort; To say, 'I am here and I understand.' "We have specialists in the field that can provide you with the therapy to treat these."

"Yes, I know. That's part of the reason I moved here. Dr. Norris and Dr. Ivy were kind enough to get a referral in, and have an appointment later next month."

"Good, good. Our therapists are unique to this clinic. They deal with epilepsy patients who have PNES. We should see positive results through this therapy."

"I'm hoping that once settled and things have calmed down; it'll make an enormous difference. I'm calmer and less stressed when I'm here. I'm not afraid like I am in BC."

"Yes, we don't want a repeat of last year, do we?" He rolled his eyes, remembering the fiasco of my marathon hospital stay.

"God, no. We move into our place on October 1. It's been a stressful year with deciding to move–waiting to sell–the move itself. Some stuff went to my brother's in Red Deer, the rest into storage. We were to stay at my brother's, but that didn't happen. We've been at my girlfriend's in Calgary. It's just been. It's been a. There's been a lot." It'd felt good to get that out. Dr. Young sat and listened, allowing me to purge myself, but it was time to leave. He was a busy man and only just returned from a conference; he had a backlog of patients to see. "Oh. One last question. Will we be continuing with the IVIG therapy?"

"No. We can rule out any autoimmune diseases. Now that we've diagnosed the non-epileptic seizures, there's no need to continue searching for what isn't there."

I was relieved, but not. It was hard to believe I had a 'mental' condition that caused seizures. It would've been easier if it were a physical issue, not emotional.

We'd said our goodbyes, and no sooner had he'd left the room when he knocked and entered again. "Ms. McClure, would you be interested in participating in a research project of mine?" Smiling, I nodded my head. It didn't matter to me what the project was. I'd already took part in most of Dr. Eastman's, and their latest on gene research.

"Of course. That's one of the other reasons for moving here, Dr. Young. I want to continue taking part in research."

"Oh. Okay, good. Have you done the gene one with Dr. Long?"

"Yes, they stole blood while I was in the SMU."

"Wonderful. I'll let Karen know. There are some forms to complete. Do you have time to sit now? And we'll squeeze you in for a follow up in six months. Bye for now." The door made a soft click as he left a second time. Moments later, a knock came and a young lady entered the room.

"Hi, my name is Karen. Dr. Young said you would like to take part..." I knew the preamble; I heard it many times over the last three years. 'We won't divulge your personal information. We'll refer to you as Patient A, blah blah blah.' We spent some time completing forms before we left.

"Where do we catch the bus, Dev?"

"It's over here, Mom." The day was bright and warm. Crystal blue skies above surrounded the glowing sun. The breeze was spreading the warmth of its rays. On all my other trips to my second home, I left by taxi; headed back to a hotel or the airport. That time, there was no need we could go by bus. It felt surreal, as if in a dream surrounded by fog. "I never thought I would see this day, Dev. Leaving Foothills by bus? What a concept."

"Yeah. Who Knew, eh?"

# Chapter Twenty-Five

## **Are You Kidding Me?**

*[Psychogenic Non-Epileptic Seizures also known as Non-Epileptic Attack Disorder (NEAD), and Non-Epileptic Seizures (NES).]*

*PNES: It's a part of my life now. I'd become so in tuned with how my head feels. Are my limbs weak or sore?–Did I feel up to going out and dealing with the hustle and bustle of other people's lives? Are the medications I'd been taking working? I'd lived each day hiding from myself–pushed away any emotions that'd tried to surface. I'd forgotten how to feel–couldn't tell the difference between thinking and experiencing. It'd been easier to ignore the pain, sadness, and anxiety. To pretend those feelings weren't there, helped made them invisible, like they'd never existed.*

*In reading Psychogenic Non-Epileptic Seizures: A Guide and Living Like You Mean It, use the wisdom and power of your emotions to get the life you really want, have taught me much. With all my feelings kept in a locked room, I became numb to where I didn't know how to feel.*

*Through awareness exercises, I learned how to identify feelings of Anger, Sadness, Happy, Love, Fear, Guilt, and Shame by 'listening' to my body. Each emotion shows itself in a physical form, from tears to increased heart rate, numbness, tension, butterflies in the stomach, tingles and breathing. They're all pieces of a puzzle we must fit together to see the picture. I should acknowledge these feelings, not ignored. Once noticed, they will move on, no longer seeking attention. By allowing myself to 'feel' again, and not worry that my emotions will overwhelm me, causing stress and the threat of seizures, I can move forward. Continuing my therapy with Dr. Harper and having easy access to my home at Foothills should make life a lot calmer. Allow me to adjust to the new me without the constant reminder of who I was—who I used to be. The old surroundings growing up heightens the sense of loss. Coming to a place with no history other than comfort and safety is a balm to the wounds I carry. I'm only known as the Linda of today, not yesterday. Some may say my move to Calgary was a little extreme and costly. But what price do you place on your health? What should your peace of mind cost?*

# PART FIVE

# Chapter Twenty-Six

## **A New Chapter or a New Book?**

### *What Now?*

I considered myself a burden to those around me, and especially my family. I felt guilty that my son had to deal with something like this so early in his life. He was 17 when that first seizure occurred. By the time he turned 21, my epilepsy had torn our lives apart. The poor kid was still finding himself. Had been breaking down the wall he erected many years ago, brick by brick. He had a social life beyond his computer screen for the first time since elementary school. Our roles had reversed. I relied on him for almost everything. He was the one I saw day in and day out, the only one I spoke to daily. Since his dad died over 12 years ago, I was both mother and father.

He grew up with no positive male role model. His grandfather ignored him, and my brother lived hundreds of miles away. Mom supported me in both the emotional and financial aspects, and when the trips to Calgary started. She was the rock I clung to with the first seizure. She got me through those months dealing with a broken system that let me down. I was in a relationship on the brink of collapse and no genuine support from home. Dev 18 was scarce, working and doing his own thing. The help she provided was a salve to my wounds. I could talk to her like no other, and she got me. The toll on her was immense. To see her baby suffering and there was nothing she could do was hard. Witnessing some of my worst seizures were devastating and horrific.

As Dr. Everly told me, my desire to hermit myself from the outside world is a form of mourning. I was grieving for that which was and can not be again — losing all that was familiar, comfortable, the status quo. Yes, I obsessed about my situation, who wouldn't? Forty-nine years without experiencing a twinge. And now, I faced a life of seizures, medication, and surgery. A lot to take in, adjust to, accept. I was dealing with a dysfunctional medical system and navigating through consults, tests, and meds. Travelling to another province was a challenge for anyone. For one whose life had unravelled and couldn't find the rope's end to tie it off, it was insurmountable.

We're on the last stretch of what will be the start of something new. I've referred to it as '*a new chapter in the book called my life.*' My life isn't over and, as far as I know, it's not ending soon. What the future holds is anyone's guess. I'm no different from the next. No crystal balls to gaze into and see what's lurking around the corner. I'm not psychic, only psycho; at least part of my brain is. It pains me to leave all that I've known. The familiar surroundings that comfort me during the emotional storms that consume me. But I'm excited to start over with a clean slate — a new province, a new home–a fresh beginning. Being a solitary person, I have no problem with spending time by myself. My son and I are two peas in a pod with that. Content in our own hobbies, we often become lost within ourselves, silent and focused on the tasks at hand.

As we get closer to our move date, I reflected over the last four years. Subconsciously, I have taken all my anger and frustration out on those around me — the loss of independence. The fear and anxiety of a future wrought in uncontrolled seizures. All the prescriptions, hospitals, and surgeries have been too much to bear. The expectations and demands I'd placed on friends and family were unreasonable. How could they know how to help when I didn't understand myself? To protect them and me from this 'new self' I had yet to figure out, I turned inward. - Surrounded by those old familiar walls– cutting off the ties that linked me to them. Only a few persisted, throwing new lines to draw me in, not allowing me to disappear. Being alone was and can be therapeutic. No expectations, no commitments, living each day as it came and went. The only interruption being doctor appointments, tests, pharmacy visits, and haircuts. Visits with others restricted on an as-needed basis. By flying solo, I focused on writing poetry, short stories, non-fiction, and contests. It had other benefits too. Able to laze about in pyjamas, watching Netflix. Falling asleep in a comfy chair with Kobo in limp hands and not worrying about makeup, throwing on worn out and ripped jeans, reliving my teen years at 53.

I don't introduce myself as being an epileptic. I take every opportunity to educate and raise awareness about epilepsy. My experiences turned my life upside down. Twisted sideways and inside out when this disease came on the scene at 49. Five years, and five surgeries later, and I'm no closer to taming this beast that lives within my brain. There's been many days and weeks that I've drowned in self-pity. Felt sorrow over what my life had become, but I've struggled on. Tapping into that Inner

Strength we all have is what's helped me keep my head above water. But. Sometimes it's easier to stay in the past. You can see it in the rear-view mirror. The movie's already played, and the credits rolled. You know how it ends. Living in the present is okay. Caught between the known and unknown provides a sense of security; you're safe for that moment in time. It's the future, what hasn't come to pass, the boogeyman under the bed — the monster in the closet that dials up the fear factor. Setting goals is hard. It requires you to look ahead and imagine a more natural life. Without dark shadows; and the demons that haunt you. It's far simpler to seek the safety of the past. To wrap it around you and cringe–the living day to day with complicated chronic disease, exhausting–torture to one's body and soul.

# Chapter Twenty-Seven

## *2020: A New Decade—Same Shit—Bigger Pile: A Pandemic*

What started out as a promising new life, full of new beginnings and firsts, came up short. People would stare at one another with suspicion, walking off sidewalks, turning away, or retreating just to avoid any contact. Staples of every day life flew out of grocery stores, leaving shelves bare for days. Online shopping and food deliveries surged, causing massive backlogs and wait times. The World faced with a global health crisis exceeding that of the Swine Flu and possibly SARS. The elderly and weak succumbed to its death grip, and hundreds of thousands died.

As I write this, my final draft hopefully, we are bracing for a second wave with the annual flu season approaching. Everyone has suffered. Lives and jobs lost, families and friends isolated, kept apart to reduce exposure. No one was immune to COVID-19 and it will take years to recoup and develop a new normal. The stress of the situation, and fears of contracting the disease, increased my stress to its highest. I became depressed, more so than I ever had. I could not control how my body and mind reacted to the pressures we were facing. Anxiety levels rose exponentially, increasing my seizure activity. For the first time, I had a seizure in the gym. I had gone down to workout in the facility provided to tenants, hadn't been on the treadmill for more than half an hour when I felt funny. My left hand wasn't functioning, it was as though I didn't know how to use it. The vision on my left became distorted, and I knew I had to go sit. I got off the treadmill, stumbled, and headed to the floor mats on the opposite side. I recall sitting with a thump. Taking my headphones off, the cord got tangled up and coiled around my neck. I believe they said. The left hand shook, the intensity increasing with each second. At one point I stood thinking I should go to the office for help. The shaking intensified. I saw movement out in the hallway, a person walking by. I yelled out. My arms flopping about like a fish out of water, crying out, saying, "I'm having a seizure. Please help. I need help." The person walked away to get help, I thought. By this time, standing became difficult as I leaned towards some gym equipment. I remained upright, for I don't know how long. I recall the water bottle slipping to the floor, the fingers of my right hand unable to hold on to it. My conscious state failed. I fell backwards, my spine slamming into an object laying on the floor. I remember feeling pain. I came to in the emergency. When the paramedics arrived, I was not responding to their questions. I'd thrown up. It took hours for the Midazolam they

403

pumped into me to release its hold and allow me to resurface. Another year I'd hoped to begin seizure free, blown. The only difference was I'd held out a week longer than in 2019.

I've been working with Dr. Harper now for a year and still find that feeling emotions you've never expressed remains difficult. Learning how to stem the storms developing under the surface takes practice and patience. Through meditation, exercise, journaling, massage, and listening to music, I've gained some knowledge and an excellent base to build on. As with life, it's a moving missile. The speed of the onset, the when, where, and how come, no different from the realities we all face. It's the players' performance that varies the effect on the audience. Over the last year, I have learned to go with the flow. Set aside my obsessive compulsiveness and let stuff just happen. I spend more time just being. My home is a tidy mess with dust and clean dishes sitting out on a drying mat next to the sink. Some days I'm not dressed until I have to leave my apartment. Recyclables collect in a bag in the hall closet and taken down every few days. Laundry done when I feel like it, and if I eat out of the fridge, deal with it!

*[This disease that resides within is tiresome but has made me stronger, I guess. I haven't given up and I'm still fighting, although my life has been broken into shards, pieces of what I used to be. Some are missing, others put back in the wrong spaces, altering my outlook on life and what it means. If there's one thing I've learned over the last 10 years, is everything happens for a reason. The decisions we make ourselves determines the path we take, or not. But when I sit down and reflect on my life and where it's been, there have been outside influences that altered my path, regardless of the decisions I made or chose not to make.*

*The people in your life help shape who you are and can make a tremendous impact on which road you travel. From the overbearing father, the friend's dad who abused me, the alcoholic ex-husband, and a toxic relationship, all tools that carved out who I am. An emotionally stunted woman, who doesn't know how to feel and whose real identity hides behind a wall of stone. No one gets in and she doesn't go out.]*

It's been a rough year. When I got the call on April 1st, I hadn't recognized the voice on the phone. It was my brother, but it could've been a stranger for all I could tell.

"Sh-she-sh-ee-e-e-es g-g-g-one."

"Jim? Is that you? Jim? Who's gone?" I remember sitting on my bed. His voice sounded like he was choking or was speaking with his mouth full.

"M-m-o-om-m-mm. M-m-mom. Mom's gone. She-e she's dead, Linda. M-mar—g-a-g-g-a-ret c-c-called me."

"What? What do you mean she's gone? I just talked to her a few days ago." I hadn't heard his response. I was locked in a bubble of silence. Chest tight, my breaths came in quick gasps—heavy and forced.

"Linda? You there? Linda?" Confused, it'd taken a few moments to return to the present—to face what he'd said.

"Yeah. Yes, I'm here. What. What. What happened? H-h-ow?" He sounded far away. A tinny voice—tired, rough, hoarse from the emotion and pain.

"K. Look. I gotta go. Sorry. But I need to go. Love ya sis."

"Bye. L-l-o-v-e you too." Silence. The tears started. I sat muttering to myself. She's gone. She's gone. My hands shook. I fell to the side. Devon stood at the door staring at me as I'd crumbled. He sat on the edge of the bed and wrapped his arms around me. He'd heard me. My voice rose as I spoke—the pain evident as the emotions of dread, surprise, anger whirled around my head, and came to a dead stop as the shock hit.

Mom had been healthy. At eighty-six, her major complaint was arthritis, a partially torn ligament in her left shoulder, knees that were stiff and prone to swelling, borderline high blood pressure, and a shadow on her lung that had disappeared. She hadn't contracted COVID - she'd gone into cardiac arrest. Not one to be a burden to her children, she had do not resuscitate orders - DNR - and the medics let her go.

### Did You Have to Die?

*you left without a goodbye. no hug and kiss or teary eye, you passed as you wished, no machines to let you exist. but did you have to die? I am hollow and lost without you here. we were close, my best friend, mother, dear. to leave me behind, left a lump in my throat, to pass on April 1st was a heartless joke. I miss you dreadfully, I need you near, the wounds are raw the pain severe. but God carried you high above, your spirit soared upon the wings of a dove. He whisked you away without a goodbye, no chance for a kiss or teary eye. your soul lives in the clouds up high, but did you have to die?*

She'd left us - went without pain - no ICU - tubes - life support - no fuss - no muss. It's been hard not having her around. No more phone calls, emails, laughter. My mother, my best friend, has gone and all I have left is memories. To help me cope, I'd write in my journal as if we were talking - letting her know what I was up to and how well me and my siblings were getting along without her.

I'm learning that I cannot control all things. That I can control what I do and what I think and how I react - sometimes. I can not predict a winning lottery ticket, the weather, or which team wins a game. I also can not predict my seizures. How long or how often. I can not know whether it's a seizure caused by my epilepsy or a psycho seizure, as I call them. There are many things I can not control and to deceive myself otherwise is disastrous. I've been living in the shadows of a chronic disease, and I've let it torment and abuse me. It's won more battles, but not the war. It has depressed me. Left me frightened, anxious, and lonely. I've had to deal with a medical system inadequate to my needs. A government unable to recognize their failings and make changes. I've spent more time in hospitals and with doctors than my friends and family. I had 28 holes drilled through my skull and my right temple cracked open three times. I know pain. I have limited use of my left hand, lost sensation in the foot and arm. And yet I still carry on.

*Epilepsy and PNES is what I have, but is not who I am. I am a Voice for Epilepsy. I speak out for others still in the shadows. I support others suffering from anxiety and depression. I share my experiences and coping strategies I hold in my toolbox. I can not control the shadows that surround me, but I can step out into the light.*

April 2021: I've spent several months now going over journal entries and hospital reports searching for clues. Now knowing I have both epileptic and non-epileptic seizures has me questioning some events over the last four years. Through therapy and reading such books as: Living Like You Mean It— Use the Wisdom and Power of Your Emotions to Get the Life You Really Want (Ronald J. Frederick, PH.D.), In Our Own Words (Mary Martiros, M.Ed. and Lorna Myers, Ph.D.) and, In Our Words—Personal Accounts of Living with Non-Epileptic Seizures (Markus Reuber, Gregg Rawlings, and Steven C. Schachter), I'm beginning to think some of my earlier seizures weren't all epileptic. It's too late to confirm or deny but is still worth looking at. Since this all started, I've needed to know why, to find a reason, a meaning for 'why me,' and why epilepsy? We'll never know. But PNES? That I could find an answer to. I just need to look in the right places. Behind walls, in boxes placed on shelves buried deep inside.

# Chapter Twenty-Eight

## **Present Day Alberta**

Our move to Calgary was a long and painful process. If I could survive the months that led up to our departure, I considered myself cured. Not in the actual sense, but mentally. I don't know what the future has in store for me—if my life here in Alberta will provide a smoother ride from years past. We're still settling in and feeling our way, discovering life in new surroundings. The weather, the people, all different from what we had, but feel right.

It's been months now without an ambulance ride to 'Foothills Chateau.' My mood has improved. It's lighter, calmer—relaxed. Not a day goes by without Dev and me venturing out, walking. Safeway is a mere five minutes away, coffee shops and restaurants close by. We love our apartment. It already feels like home. Our view includes Foothills in the distance. A constant reminder that help is not far away and my 'family' is close.

Devon still calls out or comes running should I drop something in the shower or another room out of his sight. Role reversal has taken on a whole new meaning to me. As the parent, it was me reacting to every sound, on the lookout for danger and protecting my spawn. That was no longer the case. 'I want to be sure you don't fall down and die,' he said when asked about the move and if he wanted to come. Out of love, the cooler temperatures, and snowy weather, plus his hate of the Canucks, spurred his decision to leave. I'm thankful for that and that I have him. I couldn't ask for a better son.

Unless new treatments become available, there isn't anything more to do. A handful of pills and therapy to calm a disturbed mind are all that's left. No more electrodes, drills, digging tunnels and scooping out brain matter. Four years of fighting the system. Of searching for answers, feeling terrified, guilty, and anxious. I've reached the end. Without a cure, I must continue as I am. Learning to adjust and change as I go. It is trying to control that which is uncontrollable and having to accept it. With therapy, they said we could contain my PNES—the fake ones, as I considered them. Once we've exorcised that demon, my fear of recurring 'psycho seizures' will diminish.

Neither Edwards nor Young thought it would have turned out this way. It was a simple textbook case, or it should have been. They gave me a 70% chance of becoming seizure free.

My life should have returned to normal. I should have returned to work and resumed driving. Pick up where I left off and move forward, ride off into the sunset. I don't know what went wrong, why I stare out my living room window at Foothills standing tall across the river. A guardian against all that ails me.

I shouldn't have had to uproot myself and move over 940 kilometres. The hospitals and doctors of BC should have the resources to help me, and others like me. They should have the support of the Health Ministry—of the Premier. But they don't. Because of that, neurologists like my Dr. Edwards are overloaded, overworked, overwhelmed—burnt out. Based on my own experiences, they don't have time to spend on cases such as mine; especially when you're not their patient.

I don't believe in reincarnation, but have often thought I pissed someone off in a previous life. Or fate playing a cruel joke, and Karma decided I'd deceived her, and this was payback. Whatever it was or is. This is my life now. The road I must travel. I keep reminding myself that nothing in life is easy. If it were, it'd be boring. One might as well be dead if the days carried on with no surprises. Being stuck in a rut is one thing. Not bothering to get out is admitting defeat.

Dr. Young's voice still echoes inside me, *'You're a mystery, Ms. McClure. Your epilepsy is becoming progressive. And we don't know why.'* And *'*You are an enigma … not uncommon to have both epileptic and non-epileptic… it's not your fault … brain can only handle so much … something going on within … a trigger you don't know exists.'

*Those* words have replayed through my mind a million times since. They're like a recording that won't and can't stop. After everything I've been through, I've stumped them. No one can figure me out. I'm a puzzle with missing pieces. A shattered glass with shards so damaged it's impossible to glue it back together.

# DIGNITY*

*Don't strip away my dignity just because I'm not as I once was That I'm not as you remember me Or what you want me to be again My mind and body have changed-not as I would have liked It has left me with the simple tasks of life to occupy my day But the heavy stuff, the juicy sink-your-teeth-into-stuff, it stole away My memory fails and I tire easily, but I've adjusted for that New and old technology has solved this for me Pen and paper, Google Assistant and Outlook They're my battery backup, my memory hub, if you will No need to treat me like a child who is seen and not heard Visible to the naked eye but invisible, deaf to the ear And please don't treat me like man's best friend Where I'm told what to do, when to do it and where I'm still here, I'm still the same as before My body is still in its physical form, my spirit still intact I may not be able to do or say all the things I have in the past But I haven't gone anywhere, I'm right here I'm still me and have my dignity*

414

# Acknowledgements

There are so many dedicated individuals I've encountered on this journey who have made it just that much more bearable. Of course, there's my family and friends who supported me as best they could during a time of emotional turmoil and the need for answers. The support of my doctors in BC, doing the best they could with the resources available to them. And the foresight to refer me to Calgary knowing I needed help now, not five years from then. The dedication and expertise of all those within the Calgary Comprehensive Epilepsy Program, a highly skilled group of specialists in epilepsy comprising neurologist epileptologists, epilepsy neuropsychologists, neuroradiologists, nuclear medicine specialists, clinical assistant physicians, nurses, EEG technologists, clinical neurophysiologists and administrative staff. Program lead Dr. Samuel Wiebe. Thank you to both Drs. Sharma and Macrodimitris for the opportunity to co-facilitate the UPLIFT program. For allowing me to contribute to being the first to launch this program in Western Canada. I'm extremely fortunate to have met you and worked with you. The support of all the nurses, doctors, and technologists of the Foothills Medical Centre Neurosciences Department, units 111 and 112. My Second Family. My Second Home.

The Members of the White Rock and Surrey Writers' Club, who with their guidance helped me publish my poems, Dignity and

Sea of Beds. And to Megan of Sana Counselling in Vancouver, where it all started with the Anne Paterson Stories on her blog. To the wonderful, exceptional writers and poets of the Alexandra Writers Centre Society in Calgary. A special thank you to Karen E. Lee, author of The Full Catastrophe and instructor whose Ramp up your Manuscript workshop and manuscript review were instrumental in the completion of this memoir. To Laurie Anne Fuhr, Multimodal Poet, author of Night Flying, and poetry instructor whose weekly Poetry Cafes have inspired me in learning new styles and never giving up. And last but definitely not least, Robin Van Eck, author of Rough and Executive Director of the Society, whose leadership and devotion to nurturing emerging and established authors to learn, expand, and create, has been invaluable. You are all talented, generous artists to whom I extend my heartfelt gratitude. To my editor, Virginia of Brilliant Fiction, your patience and guidance in sculpting this newbie to produce a polished piece of work. I thank you. For answering my hundreds of questions, oft repeated. I thank you. And, finally, a big thank you to the Epilepsy Association of Calgary. The dedication of these individuals to the thousands of epilepsy sufferers in Southern Alberta is second to none. Thank you. Thank you for all that you do for our community. You are all angels and a blessing to us all.

*Dignity* *\*Published in Riverbabble, Bloomsday Summer Issue #33\*\**

*Sea of Beds* *\*Published in Riverbabble, Winter Solstice Issue #34\*\**

*\*\*Republished in* Medium.com—Defuncted, A Collection of Abandoned Things, May 6, 2022.

*[Riverbabble was an online literary magazine established in 2002 and was declared defunct in March 2020].*

*[I wrote both Dignity and Sea of Beds under the pen name Anne Paterson.]*

# Resources and Other Stuff

https://epilepsycalgary.com/

https://cumming.ucalgary.ca/departments/dcns/programs/the-calgary-comprehensive-epilepsy-program

https://www.epilepsysociety.org.uk/non-epileptic-seizures

https://www.ilae.org/news-and-media/clinical-research/mortality-in-patients-with-psychogenic-nonepileptic-seizures

https://www.epilepsy.com/living-epilepsy/seizure-first-aid-and-safety

https://www.neurosymptoms.org/not-imagined/4594358022

https://www.epilepsy.com/article/2014/3/truth-about-psychogenic-nonepileptic-seizures

https://www.nonepilepticseizures.com/epilepsy-psychogenic-NES-Markus-Reuber.php

https://www.leg.bc.ca/content/hansard/40th6th/20170307am-Hansard-v43n1.pdf

https://armchairmayor.ca/2017/03/07/on-the-ledge-we-are-funding-more-mris-than-ever-before/

https://www.auntminnie.com/index.aspx?sec=ser&sub=def&pag=dis&ItemID=116809

https://www.dotmed.com/news/story/36047?mobile=0

# Epilepsy Fact:

There are over 40 different seizures ranging from the better known grand mal, to focal aware, focal unaware, and all those in between. Epilepsy is unique to each individual, as widely varied as the seizures themselves. For more information on the various types, visit the Canadian Epilepsy Alliance website:

https://www.canadianepilepsyalliance.org/about-epilepsy/types-of-seizures/

# PNES Fact:

It wasn't that long ago that doctors referenced these as 'pseudo-seizures', and prior to the 80s referred to as 'hysteria'. Even today, some in the medical profession still use the outdated term pseudo-seizures accusing patients of faking them, or looking for attention. Psychogenic Non-epileptic Seizures PNES: also known as Functional Neurological Disorder FND, Non-epileptic Attack Disorder NEAD, Non-epileptic seizures NES, amongst others. For more information, check out the PNES website at the link below.

https://www.nonepilepticseizures.com/

# Linda's Bibliography List

## EPILEPSY BOOKS:

1. Epilepsy Explained: a book for people who want to know more, by Drs. Markus Reuber, Steven C. Schachter, Christian E. Elger, and Ulrich Altrup.
2. Seized: Temporal Lobe Epilepsy as a Medical, Historical, and Artistic Phenomenon by Eve LaPlante.
3. Patient HM: A Story of Memory, Madness, and Family Secrets by Luke Dittrich, grandson of the surgeon who operated on patient HM.
4. A Mind Unraveled, A True Story of Disease, Love, and Triumph by Kurt Eichenwald.
5. Beyond My Control: One Man's Struggle with Epilepsy, Seizure Surgery & Beyond by Stuart Ross McCallum.
6. Surviving Wonderland Living with Temporal Lobe Epilepsy by Sharon R. Powell.
7. Web was Woven: Epilepsy and Depression by Sonny Chase.
8. Unashamed and Unafraid by Allison Hegedus.

# PNES BOOKS:

1. In Our Own Words by Mary Martiros, M. Ed., and Lorna Myers, Ph.D.
2. In Our Words by Markus Reuber, Gregg Rawlings, and Steven C. Schachter.
3. Psychogenic Non-Epileptic Seizures: A Guide by Lorna Myers, Ph.D.
4. View From The Floor by Kate Berger.
5. The Color of Seizures: Living with PNES by Kate Taylor and Jeffrey Underwood, RN.
6. Lowering the Shield—Overcoming Psychogenic nonepileptic seizures by John Dougherty.

# OTHERS

1. Living Like You Mean It, Use the Wisdom and Power of your Emotions to get the Life you Really Want, by Ronald J. Frederick, Ph.D.
2. What Happened To You, by Oprah Winfrey and Dr. Bruce D. Perry.
3. Remember, The Science Of Memory And The Art Of Forgetting, by Lisa Genova.

# AUDIBLES. CA.

Habit for Good Sleep Podcast, 21 Days of Meditation, Sleep; Meditation for mornings, Sleep; Bedtime stories, Sleep; 101, And so many other personal development podcasts, etc. available for free to members.

# About the author

*Linda grew up in Surrey, BC. Her career in the financial services industry from 1985 to 2015 abruptly ended with her epilepsy diagnosis. A single parent of an amazing son, she pulled up stakes and left her hometown of over 50 years to get the care she needed.*

*Her love of poetry began in her teens, developing into journalling, her memoir, and her blog. https://annepaterson.com/*

*Her poetry, written under her pen name Anne Paterson, has appeared in Riverbabble, Medium.com, the 2019, 2020, 2021, and soon to be released 2022, Poetry Marathon Anthologies, and Issue #9 of Wishbone Words.*

*Linda volunteers at Foothills Medical Centre in their Peer-to-Peer Support Program in the Seizure Monitoring Unit and co-facilitates the UPLIFT program offered through the Epilepsy Association of Calgary.*

*She currently lives in Calgary with her son, Devon, and their cat, Coco.*

*There's nothing better than spending time with a stranger, sharing the intimate bits and pieces of lives gone awry. The camaraderie of struggles is similar, yet worlds apart. There's nothing better than understanding the physical pain and mental anguish of waking in unfamiliar surroundings, bruised and battered, aching and sore. The experiences no one gets, not even family or friends. There's nothing better than the sympathy derived from knowing and feeling as the other has done. The silent stares, finger pointing, bullying and ridicule. There's nothing better than the telling of stories, the frustrations, the anxieties, the good days and the bad. The scars we share, the suicidal thoughts and depression. There's nothing better than meeting new people, expanding the circle of community around us. The solidarity of allies fighting for control. There's nothing better than giving of oneself to support and comfort another suffering in a darkness not of their doing. The reaching out to another just as scared and lonely. There's nothing better than being there, a part of a journey no one wishes to take, a trip along a winding road of fear, grief, and sadness. The resigned feelings of a hopeless future, a life without meaning or focus. There's nothing better than to talk, to cry, to vent and shout out loud rage against an unfair sentence, a life in constant turmoil, with no happy ending. There's nothing better than a friendly face, a friendly voice, a caring stranger, a knowing stranger, the empathy of a fellow warrior. There's nothing better than a selfless act of giving, listening, supporting those who now walk where you've trod, seeking answers to questions you've already faced. There's nothing better than... someone who 'gets' me.*

Manufactured by Amazon.ca
Acheson, AB